FEELING DIZZY

FEELING DIZZY

UNDERSTANDING AND TREATING VERTIGO, DIZZINESS, AND OTHER BALANCE DISORDERS

Brian W. Blakley, M.D., Ph.D.,
and Mary-Ellen Siegel, M.S.W.

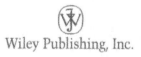

Wiley Publishing, Inc.

To order books or for customer service please, call 1(800)-CALL-WILEY (225-5945).

Library of Congress Cataloging-in-Publication Data available
ISBN 0-02-861680-4

Manufactured in the United States of America
10 9 8 7

To my wife, Joan, and my children, David, Christopher, and Laura, for their support, understanding, and sacrifice toward this book and "other projects."

B.B.

In memory of Samuel Kulkin, M.D., a leader in otolaryngology. He loved his young patients and adored his grandchildren, Betsy, Peter, and Vicki. His professional contributions made this a healthier world for the great-grandchildren he would have loved so much: Matthew, Joshua, Samantha, Hannah, and Elizabeth.

M.E.S

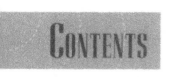

Contents

Acknowledgments

I wish to acknowledge the contribution of thoughtful clinicians and researchers who do human and animal research and wrestle with the complexities of dizziness on a daily basis. For their personal influence, I thank Drs. John H. Anderson, Murray Morrison, Michael Paparella, Hugh Barber, and Julian Nedzelski.

B.B.

Thank you to all those who support my professional endeavors: my family as well as my friends and colleagues in the Department of Community Medicine (Social Work) at the Mount Sinai School of Medicine. I am especially grateful to Drs. Helen Rehr, Gary Rosenberg, and Susan Blumenfield.

M.E.S.

FEELING DIZZY

PART I

Dizziness: What Does It Mean?

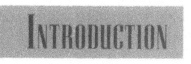

You know what it's like to be dizzy. As a child you probably experienced it when you stepped off a whirling carousel or any one of the many rides in an amusement park. Some people get dizzy looking down from heights, others every time they set out to sea. Even astronauts, trained to compensate for such conditions, often suffer temporarily from feelings of dizziness.

People often interchange the terms dizziness and vertigo, but to physicians they have different meanings. Vertigo is a form of dizziness, but dizziness is actually an imprecise term used by people to describe an assortment of feelings such as "going around in circles," faintness, giddiness, light-headedness, or unsteadiness.

In order to describe these feelings more precisely, we have defined and categorized them in the following manner:

- Vertigo: feelings of spinning or whirling
- Mild turning: the sensation of turning (but not spinning or whirling)
- Imbalance: the state or sensation of swaying or wobbling or feeling giddy; light-headedness
- Near-fainting or fainting: losing consciousness

When you are dizzy, you feel as if you can't stand straight or keep your balance. This often accompanies a bout of flu or some other virus. Staying in bed or just taking it easy, climbing stairs while carefully holding on to the banister, and perhaps avoiding driving may be all that is necessary until the dizziness clears up.

Many people also feel dizzy when they get up too quickly from a chair, jump out of bed to turn off an alarm, or rush to check on a crying child in the next room. The sensation passes quickly, especially if they sit down for a minute. Remembering to get up more slowly in the future will often solve this transitory problem.

Dizziness may also be associated with fainting, and can precede it. This loss of consciousness may follow a feeling of light-headedness, muscle weakness, and difficulty, then inability, to stand up. Fainting is usually caused by an inadequate amount of oxygen reaching the brain. It can occur during a mild illness, emotional stress, or sudden change in temperature or body position.

Vertigo, the sensation that the world is spinning—or you are—often follows a real spinning experience. One good example is the lingering illusion of motion after being spun around during a game of pin the tail on the donkey or after a ride on a carousel.

All of these feelings of dizziness, light-headedness, and vertigo emanate from the vestibular system, the collection of neural elements that work together to detect movement and position. These elements consist of the brain and the parts of the inner ears that are motion sensors. The vestibular system tells us where we are with respect to gravity and whether or not we are moving. It contributes information to the brain to allow proper balance so we can stand or walk without falling down.

Other body systems are not actually a part of the vestibular system but an important adjunct to it. These include vision, muscle tension, joint position, and touch. They contribute important information to the brain to help us keep our balance. The brain uses amazing speed and accuracy to sort out all the information it receives, then to send out instructions to the various muscle groups in the limbs, eyes, and neck to make the correct movements. In some of the examples of dizziness and vertigo described previously, the brain receives faulty information and the person feels off-balance. As soon as a correction is made by the brain, the normal feeling of balance will be restored.

For about 76 million Americans, vestibular disorders cause more than a passing problem. More than 5 million of them visit their doctors each year because vertigo is seriously interfering with their ability to work or to enjoy leisure-time activities. These people may be suffering from one or more of the conditions that cause severe or chronic dizziness or vertigo. Other individuals experience sudden, recurring dizzy spells that last only for a few minutes or several weeks. This book was written for all of these people.

We will explain how you keep a sense of balance, what can go wrong, what can be done by physicians, and what you can do to help yourself.

Even if you suffer from severe dizziness or vertigo, there is a good chance you will find help and hope from these pages, and that your life will get back on-balance.

The Balancing Act

When things are going normally, we never think about keeping our balance. We just assume that we will walk along without falling, unless we bump into something or our ankle twists. And yet anyone who has watched a baby beginning to walk, observed a preschool child standing precariously at the top of a slide, or seen a circus performer on the high wire is aware that balance is a learned skill.

In addition, balance is a reflex. If we step off a curb that we hadn't noticed, we may start to stumble, but somehow we get ourselves straightened up and are on our way again. This reflex is the result of the way our entire balance system works together in a complex but automatic interaction of all its parts. This balance system consists of the brain; the eyes; the skin, muscles, and joints of the body; and the *vestibular system* found in the inner ears.

The Complex Balance System

How does this balance system work? You could liken the intricate balancing act to a military complex or a factory. The brain represents "operation central command."

The High Command

The *brain stem* (the portion of the brain that performs motor, sensory, and reflex functions, and from where the cranial nerves of the brain mostly arise) represents the general or chief executive working out of a central command station. All orders emanate from here, and everything that happens within the complex or factory is reported back to the chief, who may at any time make changes depending on the information received. As powerful as a general or chief executive is, the president or chair can often veto or override orders. We might think of the *cerebral cortex* as supreme commander, the thinking part of the brain. It can generate commands to eyes and muscles, but the brain stem issues the actual orders.

From where does the brain receive this information? Some of it comes through the eyes—the lookouts or marketing experts—that report what's going on outside the factory. The muscles and joints are something like the clerical or support staff. They know their job and do it almost automatically, but they still need orders from the top. In addition, their activities are monitored carefully, usually not directly by the chief but rather by middle managers or go-betweens who send regular reports to the chief. In our balance system, the muscles and joints send continual messages and reports to the spinal cord and brain. These messages travel by way of nerve impulses from sensory receptors or special nerve endings within them and on the skin.

The Soldiers

A major part of the balance system is the vestibular system, located within the inner ears. This is a two-sided complex series of passageways and chambers that functions like a line of factory workers or a platoon. If one or more people make a mistake or if the machinery is not working right, the whole project is affected. Naturally, it won't take long for these troubles to reach central command.

The brain, led by its chief, the brain stem, tries to adjust for errors within the balance system, and it often succeeds. Even when our eyes send a wrong message, our knee buckles just as we descend a flight of stairs, or when our vestibular system goes off kilter because of an illness or other problem, our brain usually compensates (i.e., we grasp the railing just in time) and we keep our balance.

Altogether, we need to remember that the balance system consists of two parts: the central nervous system (brain and spinal cord) and the periphery (ears, eyes, muscles, and joints).

The Brain's Role in Balance

The brain provides an awareness of the position of our head and body in relation to gravity and objects in the environment. It is also responsible for producing those reflexes needed to keep our equilibrium. Information coming into the brain via impulses traveling along the vestibular nerve from our ears, eyes, muscles, and joints is constantly being updated. If some information is missing, inadequate, or incorrect, the brain has to rely on other information to coordinate balance.

For instance, if we get out of bed at night in a familiar room, we may not be able to depend on our eyes to locate ourselves. Instead, we use past experiences—for example, remembering there is a small step near the bathroom—and use our hands to guide us along the hallway. Thus, the brain gets information that keeps us balanced and out of trouble. However, eyes, ears, muscles, and joints sometimes send out information to the brain that is inadequate or even incorrect because of advanced age or various health problems. This means the brain is unable to create an accurate internal map.

Still, many people with these problems function well and manage to keep their balance. For reasons not fully understood by medicine, they are fortunate enough to have a brain that compensates for deficiencies. The brain, aware that it has received some faulty information, sends messages to the muscles telling them to be careful. Thus, we take smaller steps and walk slower in the dark, knowing that our "map" is not getting reliable messages from our eyes. Still, we may falter because of an incorrect interpretation of our map, and it is entirely possible we will fall flat on our faces.

The brain and its subdivisions decide on the correct position and movement of the head, neck, spine, legs, arms, eyes, and all other muscles of the body. The muscles move the body under the control of the brain, and the nerves act as wires between the brain and the muscles. All of this helps us to stay oriented: in other words, in balance. The brain stem, which is responsible for this awesome task, receives input from, and sends output to, two other areas of the brain: the *cerebellum*, which is responsible for coordination, and the *cerebral cortex*, the thinking and conscious part of the brain that is influenced by memory and learned information, whether from practice (experience) or knowledge. For instance, even if we don't stop to think about it, we have learned that it's a good idea to hold on to a banister on a steep flight of stairs. And through practice, we know to shift our weight to keep from falling when we ride a bicycle.

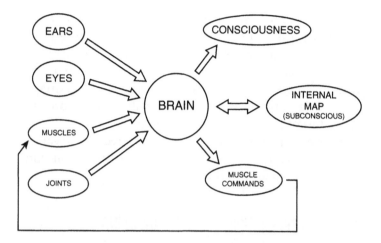

Figure 1.1   The brain creates an internal map of the world in relation to the body. It constantly upgrades the map based on information coming in. It uses the map to send control signals to the muscles of the body to cope with changes as they occur. Most events are not apparent to our consciousness.

Collecting Information

The speed and accuracy with which the brain stem collects all the information is truly amazing. The brain, like any central command, still must depend on the accuracy of the input it receives from other members of the team (the ears, eyes, muscles, and joints), as well as on its own efficiency.

Many people who have deficiencies in this receptor/processing system, the *proprioceptive system*, are prone to falls. Perhaps it is a lifelong problem and they will always be a bit clumsy. Wisely, however, they often learn to be more careful than many of their friends with more efficient systems, and can successfully avoid problems most of the time. Others may have an illness that results in delivery of incomplete information to the brain. Many elderly people gradually develop some dysfunction in their proprioceptive system, which can lead to occasional or frequent falls. (In later chapters, we will discuss more fully the causes of proprioceptive dysfunction.)

Information about movement is gathered by the various receptors in the body and processed in the spinal cord, which then relays it to the brain.

When There's a Problem with the Brain

If there is something wrong with the brain—the result of some condition or disease—our reflexes are slow and the control of balance deteriorates. All parts of the brain must work together to ensure rapid, accurate processing so that central command can send out the appropriate messages to the muscles of the body. Damage to the brain can cause muscle weakness or coordination problems that may produce feelings of imbalance.

When any one particular area of the brain is damaged, there may be localized deficits in the particular part of the body controlled by that area of the brain. Many of us know someone who has suffered a mild stroke that affected just one side of the body, for instance. With rehabilitation and time, these people often recover partial or total function.

It is worth mentioning here that chronic imbalance is usually *not* due to a localized brain deficit. Instead, the imbalance and a vague sense of dizziness may be the symptoms of a generalized reduction in brain function. A turning sensation can be caused by a stroke that involves the area of the brain where the vestibular nerves enter. However, with a stroke there will be other deficits as well, such as loss of temperature sensation or some numbness or muscle weakness.

We will keep our balance if everything is working right in the brain *and* if the input to the brain is correct and consistent. Signals to the brain that are too numerous or too confusing can result in dizziness.

Visual Input

The eyes are indeed our windows to the world, so it is no wonder that they give the brain much-needed information. But when they give us too much faulty information, we become confused, are unsure of where we are, and consequently are thrown off-balance.

Like a camera, the eye also has a lens through which light passes before focusing on the retina, the thin, light-sensitive film that lines the inside of the eyeball. There a chemical reaction takes place in which an image is briefly recorded, much as it is recorded on the film in a camera. These images are transmitted to the optic nerve at the back of the eye by means of cells called cones and rods (the two most important types of cells in the retina because they sense light). When the optic nerve receives these images, it transmits the messages to the visual centers of the brain. These messages aid in balance.

The Optokinetic and Pursuit Systems

Certain reflex eye movements are related to balance function; some are conscious and some are not. Two of these visual reflex systems are particularly important to balance function: the *optokinetic* and *pursuit systems*.

The optokinetic system is a basic or primitive reflex that causes the eyes to move when the field of view moves. Imagine you are sitting on a train that is moving through a station. You look out of the window, convinced that the station is moving—not you. That is the message that your eyes are giving your brain. Other parts of the balance system are telling your brain that *you* are moving and the station is still. These conflicting messages will throw some people off-balance but not others, depending on the efficiency of one's own personal balance system and its control by the brain.

The pursuit system is one that keeps vision fixed on an object when it moves slowly across your field of view. The whole visual field does not move. You are able to follow a bird flying in front of you, or perhaps sit in the train station and watch a distant train slowly pull out. The key feature of pursuit eye movements is that they are smooth and continuous. If you choose to follow the bird or the train past the comfortable position of the rotation of your eye, you will have to move your head. This system is a voluntary one: we decide whether or not to follow the moving object, which is not the case with the optokinetic system.

Optokinetics can also explain why a 360-degree movie screen depicting an amusement park ride can make us dizzy; our eyes tell us we are moving while the rest of our balance system says we are standing still. These conflicting messages confuse our balance system.

The Muscles, Joints, and Skin

There are about 650 muscles in the human body; each one is made up of elastic fibers that expand and contract, producing movement at the joints. The joints connect the various 206 bones in the body and are cushioned with a layer of cartilage that absorbs some of the shock or weight involved in movement. Joints also contain synovial fluid as well as a membrane, a protective casing called the capsule, and bands of fibrous tissue called ligaments that bind the parts of the joint together. Each of these muscles and joints has sensory receptors and can also send messages along neural pathways to the brain.

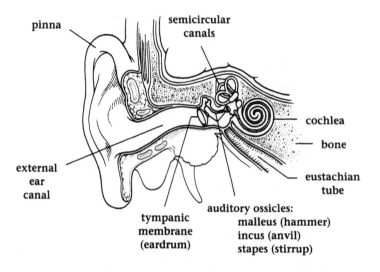

pinna

semicircular
canals

cochlea

bone

external
ear
canal

eustachian
tube

tympanic
membrane
(eardrum)

auditory ossicles:
malleus (hammer)
incus (anvil)
stapes (stirrup)

Figure 1.2 Cross section of the ear. Note that the cochlea and semi-circular canals are encased in bone.

The skin, our body's largest organ, protects the internal organs, helps to regulate temperature, and prevents dehydration. It also has pressure receptors that send messages to the brain. Especially important are the receptors on the feet and buttocks that inform the brain what part of the body is down and touching the ground.

Thus, even though you aren't conscious of it, your brain knows what your body is doing, and can send various parts of the body orders—all in the service of keeping you balanced.

Some messages or impulses may be more important than others in keeping you balanced. For instance, the impulses that come from the neck convey which way your head is turned, and those that come from your feet and ankles let the brain know the movement or pitch of your body in relation to the surface on which you are standing. The brain compensates for some of the foolish positions in which most people place themselves—turning around too far to watch a movie star walk by, or suddenly getting off an escalator without looking—so they don't land on their faces or their behinds! That is because the "chief" in the brain has over-ridden the information that the muscles or joints passed on. Other times, of course, it is the very information that the muscles and joints send that keeps you upright despite the fact that your eyes have deceived you.

When someone suffers from an illness that seriously af-fects the muscles or joints, that person may have problems with balance despite the best efforts of the brain to com-pensate for faulty information.

The Ears: An Important Role in Balance

The ear has two main functions: hearing and balance. Structurally, it is divided into three parts: the outer, middle, and inner ear.

The Outer Ear

The outer ear extends from the pinna or *auricle*, the carti-laginous portion protruding from the side of the head, to the eardrum. The outer ear canal is a passageway about $1^1/_4$ inches long that ends at the eardrum. Within the outer ear canal are wax-producing glands and hairs that protect the middle ear. The outer ear's function is to funnel and deliver sounds to the middle ear.

The Middle Ear

The middle ear reaches from the eardrum to the bone of the skull. It is an air-filled space or cavity that also contains *ossicles*, the bones of hearing. The eardrum is on one side of the middle ear, and the bone overlying the inner ear is on the other. The bones in the middle ear conduct sound vibrations, carrying them to the inner ear through the oval window, where they are processed into signals that the brain recognizes and identifies. There is a narrow tube, the *eustachian tube*, that slants down from the air space in the middle ear to the back of the nose. This passageway is usually closed, but when we swallow or yawn, it opens, allowing an exchange of air that equalizes the air pressure within the middle ear and the air pressure outside. Sometimes when we are on an airplane or in an elevator, this pressure can become temporarily imbalanced between the two sides of the eardrum.

The middle ear can also sometimes become filled with fluid, providing an environment for the growth of bacteria. A dysfunctional eustachian tube is thought to be the main cause of middle ear infections.

The Inner Ear

The inner ear is rightfully named the *labyrinth*, for it is a complex system of chambers and passageways. It is encased in an odd-shaped, complicated bone called the *temporal bone*, one of the many bones of the skull. The inner ear (Figure 1.4) contains two major parts. One is the *cochlea*, the portion of the inner ear that functions in hearing. The other is the *vestibular apparatus*, sometimes called the peripheral vestibular system, the vestibular organs, or vestibular structures. It is associated with balance and orientation and is adjacent to the cochlea, connected by a common *membranous labyrinth*. In this membranous labyrinth there is a network of three fluid-filled, membranous (i.e., made up of a thin layer of tissue), semicircular ducts suspended within the bony semicircular canals of the inner ear. Because of this connection, any disease that affects one area of the inner ear may affect others as well. And because of both the anatomical connection and the manner in which fluids easily move between the hearing and balance part of the ear, hearing and balance are often interdependent.

THE COCHLEA: THE HEARING PART OF THE INNER EAR. One opening to the cochlea is called the *oval window*. The oval window is filled by the *stapes* bone, one of three ossicles, or small bones of hearing. The other two ossicles are called the *malleus* and the *incus*. The malleus is attached to the eardrum as well as to the incus, and the incus is attached to the malleus and stapes. When the eardrum vibrates, these ossicles vibrate, conducting sound to the cochlea.

Another opening in the cochlea is called the *round window*. It vibrates in the opposite direction of the oval window, permitting a minute flow of fluid in the cochlea that allows transmission of sound by way of vibrations.

After sound waves strike the eardrum, they pass through the bones of the middle ear and then through the oval window into the inner ear. In the cochlea, the sound waves vibrate special cells called hair cells. Hair cells produce electrical impulses that are dispatched to the brain by way of the auditory nerve. There the nerve impulses are interpreted as sound.

The cochlea, which is shaped like a snail's shell, contains rows of hair cells. It is filled with two kinds of fluid, *endolymph* and *perilymph*; alterations of pressure or chemical composition of endolymph and perilymph cause certain forms of dizziness. These fluids contain potassium, sodium, and other chemicals. Despite their importance in maintaining equilibrium, the total volume of both fluids in one ear is about one-half to three-quarters of a milliliter, or just over a tenth of a teaspoon.

Endolymph flows gradually through the membranous labyrinth and down the *vestibular aqueduct* into a sac just

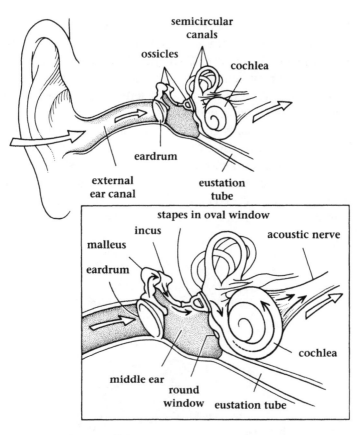

Figure 1.3 Processing and transmission of sound. Vibrations of the air are conducted to the cochlea where the hair cells change the sound energy into nerve impulses.

behind the inner ear. This sac is embedded in the fibrous tissue that surrounds the brain. Here, the liquid is absorbed into the spinal fluid that bathes the brain. Perilymph from the inner ear flows down the *cochlear aqueduct* to connect with the spinal fluid surrounding the brain. Changes in the flow, pressure, and chemical composition of the liquids from the inner ear have been thought to cause specific forms of dizziness such as *Ménière's disease*.

THE VESTIBULAR APPARATUS: THE BALANCE PART OF THE INNER EAR. The cochlea and the vestibular part of the ear are connected by channels. The function of the vestibular apparatus or system is to maintain equilibrium and balance. It consists of two types of sense organs, the *otolith organs* and the *semicircular canals*.

The otolith organs consist of one structure that senses vertical motion of the head and another that senses forward and backward motion of the head. Crystals of calcium carbonate (otoliths) are embedded on a gel. Tiny hairs from special cells called hair cells protrude into the gel from below. The otoliths act as weights, causing the hairs to bend

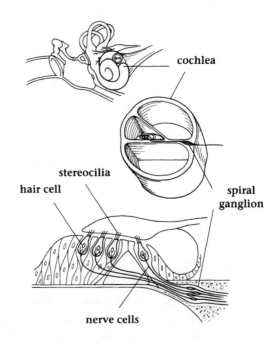

Figure 1.4 Cross section of the cochlea. This is the part of the ear responsible for hearing.

according to gravity. This mechanism allows the brain to detect the direction of gravity and help the otolith organs maintain balance.

The gelatinous mass and otoliths together are called the *otolithic membrane*. Each ear contains two otolith organs, which are oriented so that they are perpendicular to each other. These are called the *saccule* and the *utricle*. The saccule is nearly vertical when we are standing, so it senses gravity best when we are upright. The utricle is almost horizontal, so that it is most effective in detecting the direction of gravity when we are lying down. Lying down brings the utricle into a direction similar to the direction of

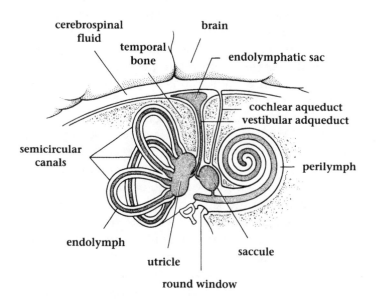

Figure 1.5 Drainage of inner ear fluids. Note that both perilymph and endolymph drain into the cerebrospinal fluid around the brain but the endolymph does so through a membrane.

gravity. Some forms of movement along a line, called linear acceleration, cause similar movement of the otoliths and so are detected by the otolith organs.

In each ear, there are three canals that follow a semicircular course. Each end of the semicircle connects to the main chamber of the vestibular system, called the vestibule. One end of each of these canals has a dilated, or swollen, end that contains a number of highly specialized sensory cells. These cells have hairlike structures that protrude into an overlying gelatinous structure called a cupula. The semicircular canals and vestibule are filled with endolymph fluid. The function of these specialized cells is to detect movement of the endolymph fluid. This is the main sensory mechanism of the vestibular system. Endolymph fluid flows along these canals most efficiently when the head is rotated in exactly the same plane as that particular canal is oriented. Rotations that are close to the plane of the canal can still stimulate the canal, but to lesser degrees.

Nature has devised an ingenious method of sensing head rotation in all three dimensions by placing one of these semicircular canals in each ear in each of three separate planes. The planes are perpendicular to each other. The geometry of the system allows it to detect rotation in any plane or combination of planes. The fact that there is a corresponding set of canals in the other ear means that there is redundancy in case injury should occur.

The hair cells of the semicircular canals do not contain calcium carbonate crystals as the otolith organs do. When you rotate your head in the same plane as a particular canal, the endolymph fluid tends to remain stationary. The cupula moves with the head because it is attached. The cupula tends to move through the endolymph. The movement of the semicircular canal in relation to the fluid causes the hair cells to bend; this in turn causes nerve cells to fire, which the brain is able to sense. Our brain interprets this as a feeling of rotation of the head. Of course, if a semicircular

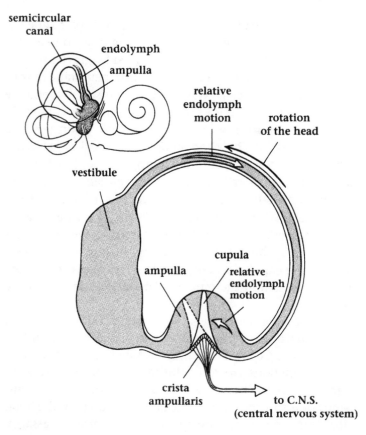

Figure 1.6 Semicircular canal function. As the head turns, the endolymph fluid tends to remain still. This "relative" motion pushes on the cupula, changing the rate of nerve impulses sent to the brain.

canal began to fire inappropriately, we would also have the sensation that we are spinning or turning. This is vertigo. Vertigo will also result if the input from one semicircular canal is missing. The brain expects the information coming from the ears to agree, or be consistent. An increase of activity in one canal should be seen with a decrease in the corresponding canal on the other side. When this symmetry is not present, due to disease for example, the person experiences vertigo.

When your head changes position in relation to gravity, either because you raise it or are moving upward in an airplane or elevator, the otoliths are pulled by gravity toward earth. This movement causes the otolith membrane to shift and bend the hair cells. When the head is still, but you are walking or moving ahead in a train or on a moving walkway at an airport, the otoliths lag behind, again bending the hair cells. This bending sends an electrical signal to the brain about how the head is moving. These signals travel along the eighth cranial nerve (the *vestibular nerve*), and when the "chief" in the brain receives this information and integrates it with the other messages it is receiving, balance is maintained. In the semicircular canals, nerve firing rates are altered by movement of endolymph, which causes pressure on the cupula. Actually, the more forceful input to the brain comes from the semicircular canals rather than the otoliths.

Both ears contain these same structures, so if one of them should become damaged or diseased, the corresponding structures in the other ear may be able to assume some of the lost functions. However, this can sometimes cause problems because the nerves will fire at different rates and thus send confusing messages to the brain. Fortunately, the brain does learn to compensate by "ignoring" certain messages. The subtleties of how the brain receives and processes this information are not fully understood. But by carefully questioning patients and selectively using tests (see chapter 3), a doctor can usually identify where the problem lies.

Integrating All the Signals

It is important to remember that the brain stem (our "chief") doesn't just receive information from all the members of the team, it also sends out a great number of memos of its own. It sends its messages by way of impulses along motor-nerve fibers to the muscles in the head, neck, eyes, legs, and all the other parts of the body that play an important role in keeping us on-balance. Much of this is automatic, but a great deal comes from trial and error, both from conscious and unconscious learning. Even those with a healthy vestibular system are often thrown off-balance, but if they are determined to learn to ride a unicycle, for instance, they will do it. Babies, whose vestibular systems are developed in only a few months, aren't able to maintain balance until somewhere between 10 and 15 months. But once they do, they quickly learn to use all the available messages received through their senses to become steadier.

On the other hand, even someone with a less than healthy vestibular system can learn to compensate for it and get back on-balance.

It is important to remember that *most* causes of vertigo are due to a problem within the inner ear. But sometimes the problem lies in other signals that are transmitted to the brain; this problem may be temporary (perhaps a new pair of eyeglasses that requires an adjustment period) or more serious and long-lasting (multiple sclerosis, for instance).

We want you to understand the varied symptoms of being off-balance so that you can answer the physician's questions accurately.

Feeling Off-Balance

Most of us have experienced an occasional bout of dizziness or even vertigo. Usually we can pinpoint the cause. Negotiating a flight of stairs with a brand-new pair of eyeglasses, trying out bifocals or a progressive lens, racing through a revolving door, getting up from bed too fast, a week-long case of the flu, excessive drinking, or taking a cough medicine with codeine—all of these can cause dizziness. The feeling is usually gone before we decide whether it is worth reporting to the doctor. Unless it's a recurring problem, we dismiss it as insignificant. And insignificant it is.

But what about a sudden, intense sense of dizziness or vertigo? Or short but repeated disrupting episodes? What do they mean?

Although most people use the word "dizziness" to describe all the uncomfortable feelings of vertigo, unsteadiness, light-headedness, and giddiness, being able to describe the differences to a knowledgeable physician can be crucial in getting a prompt and accurate diagnosis and appropriate treatment.

It is important to keep in mind that dizziness, *by itself,* usually clears up without treatment. Give it time. If the symptoms are not severe and are not keeping you from your usual activities, you may be able to wait a few weeks before visiting a doctor. Call your primary care physician (family practitioner or internal medicine specialist) if you are worried. If you describe the symptoms clearly enough, he or she may be able to reassure you.

Acute and Chronic Dizziness

When dizziness develops suddenly and the symptoms are severe but lasting just a short time, it can be a frightening experience. This acute dizziness may consist of vertigo with a whirling or spinning sensation. Some people suffer from repeated spells of acute dizziness. Generally, a problem in the ear is the cause.

Chronic dizziness, in which the symptoms are prolonged and usually of lesser magnitude than the acute kind, may produce a feeling of imbalance or floating. Most of us have experienced this type of dizziness when suffering from the flu. Many women report that menstrual cycles or, later, hormonal replacement therapy or menopause seem to be associated with dizziness. Sometimes, such dizziness is the sign of an underlying illness and it should be evaluated by a physician.

Seeing a Physician

It is likely that your primary care physician sees many patients who experience dizziness, because it is a common disorder that accompanies many different conditions. This doctor should be qualified to decide whether or not you need to see a specialist, and if so, which kind. If you have hearing loss, ringing in the ears, or other ear-related symptoms accompanying your off-balance experiences, your primary care doctor will probably recommend an *otolaryngologist* (ear, nose, and throat doctor). If you have severe headaches or neurological symptoms, including localized muscle weakness, blackouts, or persistent double vision, a neurologist should evaluate you. If some underlying illness such as heart disease, blood pressure problems, or cardiovascular illness is at the root of your symptoms, your primary care physician might suggest a cardiologist for a consultation or perhaps for ongoing care. Whoever you see will probably ask you the following questions:

- What does the off-balance episode feel like?
- When did you have the first episode?
- Do you recall having similar but perhaps milder episodes before the one that made you decide to seek medical attention?
- How often do you have these "spells"?
- What usually precedes the experience? Is it bending over, turning your head in a particular direction, driving or being a passenger in a car or other vehicle (especially if it hasn't been a problem before), rolling over in bed on one side or the other, or eating a particular food?
- Are there any other symptoms that occur before, simultaneously, or afterwards: pressure or fullness in your head, headaches, pressure or fullness in your ears, poor hearing, pain in your ears, ringing in your ears, double vision, any feelings of nausea or impending faintness?
- Is there anything that seems to make the symptoms less severe?
- Before the onset of the problem—even if it was a long time ago—did you fall, have an injury to your head, or become involved in a car accident:
- Were you or are you taking any medications, including nonprescription drugs and "recreational" drugs?
- Do you drink coffee, tea, or cola with caffeine: If so, how much?

- Do you eat foods that have a high salt content? Do you cook with salt or add it at the table?
- Do you drink alcohol, including wine and beer? If so, how much?
- Have you ever been diagnosed with diabetes, cancer, stroke, or heart disease?
- Do you have allergies?
- Prior to your symptoms, did you fly in an airplane (especially a small plane that lacked pressure equalization)?
- Have you gone scuba diving?

Defining Terms

It is important to describe your symptoms accurately. The following discussion will provide you with a clearer understanding of your condition and the terminology needed to explain it to your doctor.

VERTIGO. Vertigo is an illusion of violent rotation, a feeling that either you or the world around you is spinning. Some people use the term vertigo to describe a sensation of tilting, rocking, or falling through space. True spinning vertigo is usually caused by a problem in the inner ear that results in conflicting information being sent to the brain.

Symptoms: Symptoms may be brief and infrequent or can last for days or weeks. Vertigo that lasts only seconds is often due to something called *benign positional vertigo* (see chapter 4). Other forms of vertigo may be mild or severe. A feeling of severe spinning is usually a symptom of semicircular canal dysfunction. The problem within that portion of the vestibular system may be temporary or chronic, recurring, and difficult to treat.

A single episode of whirling vertigo and inability to walk is frightening but is also likely to get better without treatment. The more severe and acute the spinning episode, the lesser the chance that stroke or any serious brain pathology is the cause.

If symptoms of vertigo are prolonged, disabling, or progressively worse, you should see a doctor soon. If dizziness is accompanied by difficulties with vision (double vision or blindness), speech, or swallowing, or involves mental confusion, an unusual type of headache, weakness of an arm or leg, or another significant problem, it is important to see a doctor immediately.

Causes: In many cases, sudden damage to one ear causes vertigo. This is because the effects of the semicircular canals dominate those of the otolith organs. The semicircular canals sense rotational head movements, and when they aren't working correctly, you will feel as if you're spinning. Eventually, though, the brain *compensates*, adjusting to the mixed messages from various parts of the balance system.

Generally, when we rotate our head to the right, the nerves to the lateral (also called the horizontal) semicircular canal on the right increase their firing rate. (These nerves are the communication line from the ears to the brain.) The brain senses that one canal has increased its rate of firing, and the corresponding semicircular canal in the other ear decreases its rate proportionally.

This is a normal movement. We don't usually experience dizziness when we move our heads because the semicircular canals give information that is complementary to that of the other semicircular canals as well as to that provided by the eyes, muscles and joints, particularly those in the neck. But if the brain receives information from one or both ears that is in disagreement with these other senses, it becomes confused. Vertigo follows.

Associated features: Severe vertigo is usually accompanied by a type of eye movement called *nystagmus*, a series of movements, that are usually horizontal. The movement of the eyes to one side is slower than the movement to the other side in nystagmus accompanying vertigo. The result: continual tiny jerks in one direction. Nystagmus can also occur in up-and-down, or oblique directions, but this is usually a more serious problem.

Vertigo is often accompanied by a number of other symptoms. If the mismatch of sensory information reaching the brain is severe, or if the person is particularly susceptible to dizziness, it is not uncommon to experience changes in pulse and blood pressure. In addition, the individual may become pale and feel clammy, sweaty, and nauseated.

Some researchers have suggested that repeated episodes of vertigo and/or motion sickness in childhood may be a precursor of migraine headaches in adulthood.

After an attack of vertigo, whether it is brief or long-lasting, many people continue to feel unstable or wobbly and describe themselves as feeling "unbalanced." The brain is trying to compensate, but until the process is complete, these sensations may persist. They will often worsen if the person moves a bit too quickly or changes direction suddenly, or if visual stimuli are too frequent or consist of abrupt changes. Older people are more likely to experience such problems even long after the original vertigo episode because the brain may compensate more slowly than in the past. Diagnosis may be complicated, especially for those who failed to report the initial episode to the doctor and have forgotten the details.

MILD TURNING. *Mild turning* describes a less severe form of vertigo, one that allows a person to walk, work, and otherwise show no outward signs of impairment. Because most of us evaluate discomfort in relation to other experiences, if you have never experienced true severe vertigo, mild turning may still seem rather upsetting to you. And indeed, it is certainly worth discussing with your physician because it is not necessarily trivial and easily dismissed.

Turning can be a sign of mild ear dysfunction. It may precede, coincide with, or follow a viral infection or bout with the flu, and usually clears up spontaneously.

Mild turning can also be a symptom of brain dysfunction or the result of a stroke or *transient ischemic attack* (TIA), a usually brief episode of insufficient blood flowing to the brain. Other possible causes include multiple sclerosis, previous head injury, AIDS, or almost any severe systemic illness.

Those who have suffered a stroke may report mild turning, but they will also have other signs of brain involvement, such as weakness of one side of the body, an inability to speak or swallow properly, or double vision. Sometimes, these other conditions are subtle and may go unreported until the dizziness forces the individual to see a doctor.

IMBALANCE, LIGHT-HEADEDNESS, AND GIDDINESS. Imbalance or unsteadiness could be described as a feeling of uncertainty about one's position, or a feeling of movement as if one were aboard a ship. If you experience either sensation, you are likely to want to grab hold of something or someone to help get your balance: you fear falling, but not because you are actually falling. Giddiness is a perception of disorientation, sometimes described as fogginess or cloudiness without a feeling of vertigo or imbalance. People often describe themselves as feeling confused, and yet they really aren't. Others say it's like an "out-of-body experience."

A continuous feeling of giddiness with symptoms such as apprehension, irritability, sweating, or a lump in the throat is in all likelihood the result of anxiety. If the giddiness is associated with ear symptoms such as deafness, *tinnitus* (tinkling or ringing in one or both ears), or discharge, it suggests an ear problem. Sometimes, all symptoms will disappear once the ear is treated.

Imbalance may be caused by a number of illnesses, such as influenza, infection, or general medical problems. Often, the imbalance is the first symptom you notice. You may have a feeling you're falling or veering to one side, or you may sense some instability. If the feeling persists, a physician will look for muscle weakness, especially if you are recovering from a stroke or demonstrate other neurological problems. Joint pain and stiffness from arthritis, especially in the neck, or a rheumatoid condition can also make you feel unsteady. Some people blame their unsteadiness on clumsiness, but if they are having trouble rising from a chair, the real reason may be weakness.

Problems with the spinal cord, including compression (something pressing on the nerves) or various traumas, can cause loss of sensation as well as weakness in the legs. Disturbances in blood chemistry or metabolism can also cause imbalance, as can ear or brain diseases and other problems with the balance system. A lesion (abnormality) that is slowly developing in the ear can also give rise to symptoms of imbalance. When an ear ailment is the cause, imbalance or other types of dizziness are often worsened by rapid head movements.

ATAXIA. Clumsiness may exist without any muscle weakness or stiffness. *Ataxia* is a term used to describe an impaired ability to coordinate movement. A number of medications can cause it, particularly anticonvulsants used to prevent seizures. Ataxia can result from poor information from the eyes, ears, or other parts of the balance system, or a disease in the brain. It can be either mild or severe, usually depending on its cause.

DIABETES. Diabetes can cause some unsteadiness. If you haven't had a checkup that included urine and blood tests for some time, you may be suffering from the disease without knowing it. The best-known symptoms of diabetes are excessive thirst and urinating large amounts; these symptoms are ignored by many people. Perhaps the first time that diabetics are aware of significant and even advanced symptoms is when they have to urinate frequently at night and find they aren't very steady as they walk around. This may be because the dizziness is a manifestation of their metabolic problem or because the disease has already caused degeneration of peripheral nerves.

ALCOHOL ABUSE. Drinking too much has long been related to physical unsteadiness and imbalance. The stereotype of the town drunk is someone staggering down the road. However, unsteadiness can result from alcohol abuse and alcoholism whether the person is sober, goes on drinking binges, or is in early recovery. Alcoholism can cause nerve cell loss and then dizziness. It can also sometimes cause a vitamin B deficiency that may lead to nerve degeneration and thus unsteadiness.

MEDICATIONS. Many medications that you take for a temporary condition cause dizziness as one of many potential side effects. You may experience this as light-headedness, not vertigo. Cough medicines and antihistamines are frequent culprits. Medicines for hypertension (high blood pressure) can produce a feeling of light-headedness or dizziness, especially early in the morning when one's blood pressure may be especially low, or when one rises suddenly from sleep or from sitting. A number of tranquilizers and anticonvulsants may cause balance problems. Another medication that occasionally causes such problems is nitroglycerin, which is used to dilate arteries in those with angina. It may be administered alone or combined with beta blockers such as Inderal. Exposure to mercury and lead compounds, as well as to organic chemicals like cleaning fluids and various solvents, can also cause feelings of imbalance. Many kinds of recreational drugs, such as cocaine, can cause these symptoms, too.

SYPHILIS. A history of untreated or inadequately treated syphilis can cause a sensory neuropathy that can affect the balance system.

CANCER. Diagnosed or undiagnosed cancer particularly if it involves the lungs or ovaries, can cause a nerve degeneration even though it hasn't spread beyond its original site. Cancer that has spread to the brain can also cause symptoms of imbalance.

AGING. Older people frequently suffer from imbalance because of changes in the brain that occur with aging. For instance, some brain cells decrease their activities or even die. This may have no effect on overall intellectual functioning, but retrieving just the right word for a crossword puzzle, remembering grandchildren's birthdays, or even writing a letter may take more time than it once did. If those brain cells needed to integrate the information arriving from the ears, muscles, and joints aren't quite up to the task, imbalance may follow. Sometimes the problem is within the inner ear itself, and may be another result of aging. Arthritis in the neck, a common condition in older people, can also cause dizziness and imbalance. The symptoms may be either episodic or relatively constant.

ANXIETY. Anxiety can also cause a feeling of lightheadedness, giddiness, or imbalance. Getting to the cause of the anxiety can be a big help in alleviating symptoms. Since there are so many causes of dizziness, it is important to be able to describe your symptoms accurately enough to help your doctor make the right diagnosis.

Fainting

Fainting can have many causes, ranging from a sudden drop in blood pressure to a reaction to medication, slow or rapid heart rate, stroke, heart attack or vascular problem, pressure on the carotid sinus (an area in the neck that when compressed can drop blood pressure and thus cause fainting), insulin reaction in a diabetic, or severe anxiety. The sensation is different from imbalance, vertigo, and mild turning, although any form of dizziness can precipitate such a reaction.

Symptoms

A definite feeling of fainting, or *presyncope,* can occur even if you don't lose consciousness. The feeling is similar to drifting off to sleep while in bed or perhaps while listening to a concert in a stuffy auditorium. Usually it comes on quickly and is brief, and you fully recover from it. However, presyncope *can* be more complex, unpleasant, and frightening. Often, it is associated with weakness or lightheadedness, and you feel as if you will fall or faint. It may be especially frightening if vision becomes dim and arms and legs feel weak and useless.

Causes

Both fainting and feeling faint usually result from insufficient blood supply to the brain. This can occur when the brain suddenly and momentarily doesn't get enough blood, and symptoms most often include a sharp and rapid drop in blood pressure accompanied by slowing of the pulse. Forceful coughing, or straining to urinate or move the bowels, can also cause this.

Some people faint or feel faint when they see something very upsetting, such as an accident or a frightening medical procedure, and their heart fails to deliver enough blood to the brain. An experience that causes anxiety or hysteria can make a person *hyperventilate*. This is a condition in which breathing becomes very deep and rapid and too much carbon dioxide is exhaled. Through a series of chemical reactions, this changes the acid/base balance in the body, which may cause dizziness and/or fainting.

Drop Attacks

A *drop attack* is often confused with fainting or feeling faint but has different causes. Most often, it occurs when muscles become weak so that a person falls down. Consciousness is not lost, and the person will remember the event, perhaps saying, "My knees just gave way," or "It seemed like the sidewalk just pulled me down."

Generally, elderly people are the ones who suffer from drop attacks. The cause is most commonly a blockage of a particular set of blood vessels in the brain and is not likely due to a muscle disorder or brain disease.

In some instances, particularly in those suffering from Ménière's disease, a disorder of the vestibular system (see chapter 4), the semicircular canals are no longer functioning and the otolith organs no longer send messages to the brain about the direction of gravity. Drop attacks, that is, sudden collapse or falling to the ground without loss of conciousness, also occur in a rare variant of Ménière's disease (see chapter 4).

Ocular Dizziness

That new pair of glasses, especially if it included a major change in magnification or was prescribed to correct *astigmatism*, can make you feel dizzy. Astigmatism is a condition in which the curve of the cornea is uneven, making it difficult to clearly focus on an object. The result is blurred vision. Sometimes, people are temporarily dizzy following removal of cataracts or a lens implant.

Learning to compensate for damage to the various parts of the balance system may be slow, particularly in older people. In instances where the magnification of new lenses is high, the part of the visual system responsible for sending information to the vestibular portion of the brain may have trouble adapting to the change. In time, compensation usually takes place.

Sometimes, when the vestibular system is severely impaired and function is absent, a condition called *oscillopsia* develops, in which there is an illusion that stationary objects are moving back and forth or up and down. The vestibular system normally reacts to movements caused by the person's heart beating and breathing, but when the system is defective, it is unable to perform normal compensation for this slight movement. Oscillopsia and the accompanying dizziness experienced can be quite disabling especially if the condition is chronic and persistent. Upon examination, nystagmus is usually noted in the early stages of this illness.

Multisensory Dizziness

Multisensory dizziness is a term that is often used when the specific cause is unknown. It describes a generalized dizziness that seems to have many causes, yet no one cause seems to fully explain the symptoms. Most often experienced by older people or by those with diabetes, multisensory dizziness can be more severe in unfamiliar surroundings. It usually improves if sensory input is strengthened by control of diabetes, correction of visual and hearing problems, or, if needed, use of a cane or walker.

Motion Sickness

Familiar to most people whose pleasant boat ride turned into an encounter with rocky seas, *motion sickness* affects some people more than others. Children are especially vulnerable to motion sickness, but they usually outgrow it. Dizziness, nausea, vomiting, and a generalized sick feeling are all symptoms of motion sickness. Generally, stimulation to the vestibular system within the inner ear as well as visual stimulation are the causes. The longer you are in a moving vehicle—a car, an airplane, or a boat—the more likely it is that prolonged stimulation of your vestibular system will cause motion sickness. Many of those who suffer from motion sickness will have symptoms for a few days or longer *after* the trip—a condition that is dubbed *mal débarquement* syndrome.

Related to motion sickness is space sickness, a condition caused by abnormal vestibular stimulation and aggravated or provoked by active head movements. Almost half of all astronauts have experienced it, and it appears to be related to the absence of gravity. Thus, most people never experience it.

Height dizziness or sickness is reported by many people who are uncomfortable when the distance between them and any stationary object becomes very large. The normal sway of the body sensed by the brain clashes with visual information that implies that the person isn't moving. It's not surprising that when you look out of a window that has a railing just outside, you may not suffer height dizziness, but when you look out of a large picture window at a low building across the street, a sensation of dizziness might occur. Some people feel so anxious in this situation that they think they suffer from acrophobia (fear of heights), but it is really only a physiological reaction of the balance system.

When you consult a physician, be sure to describe your symptoms as we have discussed them in this chapter. Keep in mind that other symptoms, as outlined on the following pages, may also be present. Don't think (or let others convince you) that your symptoms are imagined or psychological, but consider the possibility that they may be partly psychological.

For instance, visual problems may cause difficulties with focusing—objects or print may seem to jump around. Lights may seem to flicker or glow. Night vision may be decreased, and you may have trouble with depth perception. Fortunately, visual problems are unlikely to cause chronic dizziness.

Hearing problems may also be related to dizziness. Hearing ability may be good one time, poor another, and you may hear distortions of sounds. You may feel uncomfortable in noisy environments, and your ears may feel full.

Along with dizziness, there may be a sense of nausea and other feelings of motion sickness, even when there is no obvious cause. You may even have some memory problems. It is not unusual to become clumsy, to have trouble walking straight, and to feel and appear uncoordinated. Headaches may occur, and you may be uncomfortable with weather changes. High altitudes may worsen your symptoms. Allergies may be related as well.

All of this can make you feel depressed and anxious because you sense a loss of control that diminishes your self-confidence and self-esteem. A physician may think that your balance problems are the result of your emotional state, not realizing that your emotional state is simply the result of your balance problems.

It is therefore crucial that you observe and report your symptoms as accurately as possible.

Finding the Cause of Dizziness and Vertigo

You've been feeling miserable. Either you are suffering from occasional bouts of dizziness or it's a chronic, never-ending condition, making you think you will never be yourself again. Don't despair, for you are already gaining control over your problems. Now that you have learned the difference between vertigo, mild turning, imbalance, syncope, presyncope, ocular dizziness, and drop attacks, you will be able to describe your symptoms accurately. You may also have a number of ideas about what is wrong. You may feel you have only a temporary problem in the vestibular system that will clear up soon with or without treatment. Or you may be afraid it is more serious.

The First Visit to the Doctor

When you visit your primary care physician, the doctor will try to rule out certain possibilities and consider others based on your history and description of symptoms. For instance, if you describe your vertigo as the world rotating, the doctor will likely conclude that the problem lies in the semicircular canals of the inner ear. If you describe a feeling of being propelled or tilting and say that when lying down with your eyes closed, you feel as if you are slightly turned or your feet raised, the doctor will probably suspect that the problem concerns the brain or the vestibular system, especially the otolith organs. These organs are related to linear acceleration or gravity.

At this first visit, you may be quickly put at ease.

When the only complaint is vertigo, there is usually no other serious medical problem. Still, there could be an underlying medical or structural cause that needs to be treated before this dizziness itself can be addressed. For this reason, the doctor will want to investigate further.

Most physicians are familiar with dizziness, but there are no rules about how they assess the condition. Unfortunately, this means that the quality of the evaluation, the selection of tests, and the physician's ability to arrive at a meaningful diagnosis vary considerably. However, a well-trained physician who is either a primary care physician or specializes in otolaryngology or neurology is not only acquainted with dizziness but knows how to do a basic evaluation.

Physicians tend to view symptoms as they apply to their own specialty or expertise. A primary care physician, such as a family practitioner or internist, will look for a number of problems, whereas a cardiologist may focus on the heart and blood vessels as possible causes of the dizziness. Neurologists may want to rule out a lesion or degeneration of the brain, a head injury, multiple sclerosis, or epilepsy as the cause. Otolaryngologists usually think of dizziness in terms of ear diseases.

The following specialists can be approached directly for an appointment, or may be suggested by your primary care physician:

- See an *otolaryngologist* if you experience hearing loss, ringing in the ears, or other ear symptoms accompanying the dizziness.
- See a *neurologist* if you suffer severe headaches, have localized muscle weakness, or experience blackouts or persistent double vision in addition to dizziness.

Any doctor you see should take a careful history of your symptoms and give you the opportunity to add information that you feel is important or relevant. Despite sophisticated technology, an in-depth history is still considered the single most important part of an examination for dizziness. Thus, the doctor you consult should first talk with you and then give you a general examination, but he or she will also administer a number of other tests that you may never have had before.

History

The physician will ask you many of those questions covered in chapter 2. This will be done to elicit answers about the kind of feeling of dizziness you experience. Is it true vertigo (the illusion or sensation that you or the room are whirling), feeling that you are about to faint, or lightheadedness?

Have you had any associated illnesses or experiences? For instance, an ear infection or trauma to the head, perhaps including the ear? The doctor will want to know if your discomfort occurs occasionally or episodically and how long it lasts. Is it continuous? How severe is it? Do you experience nausea and vomiting at the same time? Are there any other ear or hearing problems?

Certainly the physician will want to know about any symptoms of central nervous system diseases. Thus, you will be asked questions regarding loss of consciousness, as well as confusion, memory loss, trouble swallowing, or any sense of numbness. You will be asked about any recreational drugs and about your alcohol consumption.

You will also be asked about any prescription or non-prescription drugs you may be taking. The doctor will be especially interested in anticonvulsants, aspirin or aspirin-like medications, sedatives, tranquilizers, and certain intravenous antibiotics, all of which can cause vestibular toxicity even in normal doses.

You may be asked if you hyperventilate. Hyperventilation means breathing too deeply, a condition that, contrary to common sense, makes you feel as if you can't get enough air. This can make you dizzy. Most often, hyperventilation is caused by anxiety.

Physical Examination

Expect a complete head and neck examination, including the nose, sinuses, and ears. Much of the exam is done with simple office instruments that will be familiar to you from other office examinations, and the rest will be done simply by palpating (touching) parts of your head and neck.

The physician will also do some neurological testing even if that is not his or her specialty: observing your walk, asking you to follow a moving object with your eyes, and examining your eyes.

You may have a basic cardiovascular examination in which your blood pressure is taken, your heart is listened to with a stethoscope, and an *electrocardiogram* (EKG) is given.

If this physician sees anything untoward, you will be sent to the appropriate specialist. If the physician does not see any problems at this time, you may be advised to wait a few weeks (unless you have already had the problem for a while). If the symptoms persist, you will be sent to one or more specialists who have an interest and expertise in treating people who suffer from dizziness.

If the physician you consult about dizziness doesn't listen to your history and do a thorough physical examination (as outlined above and below) but just sends you for tests, *see a different doctor!*

A medical examination, either at the office of your primary care physician or a specialist, will probably include the following:

CARDIOVASCULAR SYSTEM. The physician may listen to your heart and to other parts of your cardiovascular system (neck, groin) with a stethoscope. Disease in the heart valves or in the carotid artery of the neck can be a cause of dizziness.

Blood pressure can offer important clues to dizziness. One of the most common types of dizziness is caused by *postural hypotension* or orthostasis. Both terms refer to a problem of blood pressure, in which the pressure drops when you stand or sit up. (Note: *Hypertension* means high blood pressure; *hypotension* indicates low blood pressure.) If you have postural hypotension, you will find that when you get up from a lying or sitting position, especially after a long period of time (such as in the morning, or after an evening of watching television in your favorite chair), you will feel faint. Generally, the sensation lessens after a few minutes, but sometimes it worsens and you may actually pass out.

Why does this happen? Visualize the blood vessels as a series of fluid-containing tubes that run lengthwise through the body. When you lie down, these tubes are horizontal, and the pressure is fairly uniform in the tubes from end to end. But when you stand up, the tubes are now vertical, forming columns of fluid (blood). The pressure at the bottom of the column (near the feet) is much greater than the pressure at the top where the brain is located. In order to drive the blood to the brain, the vessels in the feet and legs must constrict. If the blood doesn't reach the brain quickly enough, you may feel faint or actually pass out.

The blood vessels are not just like your common garden hose containing water; they contain valves and other local control mechanisms to increase the blood pressure and deliver blood to the brain. But since humans, complex as they are, are not perfect machines, some of us suffer from postural hypotension. Our blood tends to pool in the lower parts of the body unless our blood vessels react and provide more blood to the brain.

Doctors can test for postural hypotension in a practical, uncomplicated way. They simply take your blood pressure while you are lying down and then again after you stand up. Some physicians have a special table that adjusts your position for this purpose. Your pulse will also be taken, usually along the thumb side of the wrist. The pulse measures the regular throbbing of the arteries caused by the successive contractions of the heart. Thus, the pulse should increase to compensate for the fall in blood pressure; feelings of faintness occur while the blood pressure falls.

Although there is some disagreement among physicians as to what constitutes an abnormal fall in blood pressure, usually either a significant change occurs, or there is almost no change at all.

To understand this process, you need to know how blood pressure is measured. You are probably familiar with the fact that blood pressure has two numbers. The *systolic* pressure is the first number given—the high number. It results from a contraction of the heart. The other number—the lower one—is called *diastolic* pressure. This is the pressure that remains between the heart contractions. A typical normal blood pressure is 120 over 80, written as 120/80 mm Hg. Any blood pressure consistently higher than 140/90 mm Hg may be considered high. Blood pressure norms vary according to age and other medical conditions.

This is how some physicians assess that hypotension is present:

- A drop in the systolic blood pressure of 20 or greater upon standing *and*
- An increase in the pulse greater than five beats per minute upon standing *and*
- A systolic blood pressure significantly below normal after standing.

If the blood pressure remains in the "high" range when you suddenly get up, your dizziness is not caused by postural hypotension.

Anyone who is taking blood pressure medications, has diabetes, or is over age 50 is particularly susceptible to postural hypotension. Some treatment for this condition is just common sense: (1) Move slowly when getting up, and don't stand up directly from a lying position. Instead, sit for a minute or two first; (2) Increase fluid intake. Your doctor may also include an adjustment to your blood pressure medication, if you are currently taking one.

HEAD AND NECK EXAMINATION. An examination of the head and neck includes the ears, which is essential because that is where much of the balance system is located. For instance, the doctor will listen for any *bruit*, an abnormal sound or murmur, in the neck. The physician may examine your mouth and tongue, listen to your voice, and ask you about swallowing. The structures of the mouth and throat are affected by the cranial nerves that exit through the base of the skull. Cranial nerve function can be impaired by tumors, strokes, or some neurological deficit. The eighth cranial nerve connects the vestibular system to the brain and then to eye movement, so it may affect balance. It is important to note that cranial nerve abnormalities are *seldom* the cause of dizziness when this is the only symptom, but the cranial nerves should be checked. If there is any pathology there, it is serious and needs prompt attention.

Dizziness is sometimes associated with various problems within the ears, such as hearing loss, discomfort from loud noises, or ongoing noise in the ear, known as tinnitus. The problems in the ear most often associated with dizziness cannot usually be diagnosed by just a physical examination of the ear. That is because the inner ear, where the vestibular (balance) portion is located, is not visible with an *otoscope*, that familiar instrument with a light, a magnifying lens, and a tip that the physician carefully inserts into the ear as far as the eardrum. The otoscope permits examination of the external ear, the eardrum, and some of the bones of the middle ear located beyond the eardrum.

OTITIS MEDIA. The otoscope can detect *otitis media*, an acute and usually painful ear infection of the middle ear. When the infection clears up, so does any related dizziness.

LABYRINTHITIS. Sometimes used as a general term for a mild problem within the labyrinth of the ear that is causing some dizziness or discomfort, *labyrinthitis* may mean different things to different people.

1. *Bacterial infection.* An infection of the labyrinth can cause extreme vertigo, nausea, vomiting, and nystagmus (jerky, rhythmic eye movements usually involving both eyes). The infection is most often bacterial, usually having spread from acute otitis media of the middle ear. All hearing in one ear may also be lost. Although these symptoms are terrifying if they come on suddenly, they may be partially treatable with antibiotics.

True labyrinthitis often results in hearing and/or vestibular deficits over the long term. Severe symptoms of dizziness usually abate within a week, but some dizziness may last up to a few months. The hearing loss is permanent.

2. *Viral labyrinthitis.* Viral labyrinthitis is far more common than the bacterial type. The symptoms of severe vertigo, made worse by head movement,

often follow a viral infection of the upper respiratory or gastrointestinal tracts. Some viruses can damage the ear before birth.
3. ***Vestibular neuronitis.*** When vertigo is acute and severe but not associated with a hearing loss or other signs, it is most often called *vestibular neuronitis* (see chapter 4). Careful examination helps differentiate between labyrinthitis and vestibular neuronitis, and even helps to distinguish these conditions from some other causes of dizziness.

Even when nothing painful or apparently acute is occurring, there is value in a thorough ear examination because impacted wax, foreign bodies in the outer ear canal, retracted eardrums, or trauma of the middle ear all may cause sensations of mild turning.

FISTULA. The doctor may do one of several simple office tests for a *fistula* (hole) in the inner ear. You will be asked to look straight ahead while the doctor presses on your ear or performs other simple manipulations. Certain positive signs, such as your eyes spontaneously turning to the side or your own observation about experiencing vertigo, will alert the physician to investigate further.

If the eardrum is intact, this positive fistula test may indicate the existence of scar tissue or bony erosion within the inner ear that is associated with a perilymph fistula, congenital syphilis, or Ménière's disease (see chapter 4).

HEARING LOSS. Many physicians will do some office examinations that screen for hearing loss. Although not a substitute for an audiogram (a carefully administered hearing test done with sounds, voices, and headphones, in a sound-barrier booth or room), tuning-fork testing can help differentiate normal from abnormal hearing. By placing a vibrating tuning fork on a solid midline surface, such as the forehead, the vertex of the skull, or behind the ear, the physician can distinguish between sensorineural and conductive loss of hearing.

EXAMINATION OF THE EYES. The physician may use the *ophthalmoscope*, a device with a light and mirror, to examine the inside of the eyes. It can help alert the physician to further investigate the possibility that vascular diseases, diabetes, or other problems exist because certain signs are evident in the eyes.

Nystagmus: Of great relevance to an examination for dizziness, the eyes can give major clues about abnormalities in the vestibular (balance) system because they often manifest nystagmus. Especially significant is a slow drift to one side and a rapid flick back. These involuntary eye movements may only appear in certain positions of the gaze, and may not be apparent to family or friends, but they will be evident to the examining physician. Like many neurological signs, such involuntary movements can alert the physician that something is wrong. They may even reveal where the trouble lies (although nystagmus in itself is insufficient to make a diagnosis). As the brain begins to compensate for the conflicting messages it is getting from the vestibular system, or as the injury or disease abates, the nystagmus begins to decrease.

The physician may then conduct the pursuit test. You are asked to use your eyes (without moving your head) to follow a flashlight, extended index finger, or object as it is slowly moved horizontally and vertically in front of you. Healthy, normal people can follow this with a smooth, continuous movement, but those with certain medical problems may have poor control of eye movement, and will use jerky movements to keep the target in the right spot on the retina.

The physician will take careful note of any nystagmus observed in an office examination. If the eyes move horizontally—or as in some diseases, in a rotatory manner—it usually indicates a problem with the ears. If the nystagmus is vertical or oblique (slanting, or any variation from perpendicular or horizontal) it suggests a problem within the brain.

The vestibulo-ocular reflex: The *vestibulo-ocular reflex* can also be tested to a limited extent in the office. This reflex consists of those eye movements evoked by stimulation of the vestibular system. This reflex normally helps keep the eyes on an object or target as the head moves. In order to look at a fixed object when moving your head, your eyes must move in the direction opposite to the head movement, at precisely the right speed. Thus, if you look at an object to your right and want to keep looking at it as you turn your head toward it, you need to make an eye movement exactly equal, but opposite to, the head movement.

Naturally, you don't think about this, since it is a reflex. If the two movements are not equal, it is because this reflex

---

You can do a simple test right now yourself that will compare your reading ability with and without vestibular input. First read this book holding it about eighteen inches from your eyes. Begin to move your head back and forth while reading the book. Increase the speed and frequency of your head movements gradually. Notice that you can read the print (if your vestibular system is normal) even though your head is moving quickly. Now, hold your head still and move the book back and forth. You are not getting any vestibular system information to help you. Notice that you cannot read the book when you move it quickly. This demonstrates that the vestibular system is important in maintaining gaze, especially at high speed.

> If your vestibular organs are not in good work-
> ing order, you will find it difficult or even impos-
> sible to read during the first part of the test,
> because your vestibulo-ocular reflex is missing. This
> causes a condition known as oscillopsia, in which
> objects seem to move back and forth. When you
> look ahead while walking, things in the horizon
> seem to bounce around. Chances are you have
> already experienced this if you try to read book
> titles while strolling down the aisle in a bookstore
> or library. You also probably noticed that you had
> to move slowly down the aisles of a supermarket
> to focus on the names of the products.

isn't working right and you will become dizzy or have
visual blurring. Such a reaction suggests to the physician
that you have a vestibular disorder. Two systems are required
for a healthy vestibular ocular reflex: the visual system and
vestibular system. The visual system helps us see the target
and follow it if it moves; the vestibular system keeps the
gaze centered.

Neurological Examination

Not everyone suffering from dizziness needs a complete
neurological examination, because this would include many
procedures that do not pertain directly to the vestibular
system. However, your physician may perform many of the
following tests in order to evaluate your cerebellar, proprioceptive, and vestibular function. Rarely are they all
needed. Expect the physical examination to vary considerably. We do want you to be familiar with some of the procedures that may be performed.

Mental Status

The examiner will ask you some questions to determine if the overall function of your brain is intact. Questions will include such things as the current date, season, and your full address. To assess memory, you will be asked to repeat any three words, then later recall these items. You may be asked to fold a paper, draw a clock, write a sentence, and do some simple arithmetic. A person with a disease or other problems of the brain may have impaired mental function as well as dizziness.

Tendon Reflexes

The physician will stimulate your reflexes by tapping your knee or ankle lightly with a rubber-tipped hammer to test peripheral nerve condition, motor nerve function, and spinal cord connections.

Sensation

Sensation is tested to determine if your peripheral nerves and central nervous system are functioning well. The doctor will brush your skin with a wisp of cotton or tissue paper, lightly poke you with a pin, or test your hearing with a tuning fork to assess the function of different nerves and their branches that involve different anatomic areas of the brain.

Muscle Strength and Tone

Muscle strength is tested by having you squeeze the examiner's fingers or push against the examiner or an object with your arms, legs, or jaw. Muscle tone is assessed by the physician moving your arm or leg, and perhaps both legs, to see if there are differences between the sides of your body. This helps determine if there are problems in the nerves that stimulate different muscle groups.

Coordination

To test the function of the cerebellum, you will be asked to do a number of tests that measure coordination. For instance, you will be asked to close your eyes and place a finger on your nose.

You may be asked to place your extended index finger on that of the physician's, close your eyes, raise that arm and index finger to a vertical position, and than return the index finger to the physician's. If you consistently deviate to one side, it is called pastpointing.

The doctor will also assess your ability to perform rapid alternating movements by having you quickly flip your hand on your thigh, first striking it with your palm down, then with your palm up.

Gait and Stance

Your gait and posture are related to coordination and sense of balance. Measuring them is an important part of the neurological assessment, because many people with abnormalities in their sensory processing system have a very difficult time walking. The doctor may watch you as you enter the room and walk to a chair. This can offer many clues. Another method is the Romberg test: You will be asked to stand with your feet together, without holding on to a chair or desk, and then to close your eyes. This helps the physician determine if vision has been keeping your feelings of imbalance to a minimum.

You may be asked to do progressively difficult tasks with your feet—some of them with your eyes closed. For instance, you must walk with one foot directly in front of the other. Vestibular problems may impair this so-called tandem walking when your eyes are open and your hands are at your side, but it is an even more sensitive test when done with eyes closed and arms folded against the chest.

Abnormal reactions to these tests can indicate that your sensors are not working properly and that somehow your brain isn't getting messages about your body's positions.

Cranial Nerves

Cranial nerve function should be tested in every patient who complains of dizziness. These nerves exit through the base of the skull, where the ears are located, and are adjacent to the portion of the brain stem where nerve impulses from the vestibular part of the ears accumulate. Thus, problems with the cranial nerves could manifest themselves as dizziness.

The physician has a number of simple tests that can assess each of the twelve cranial nerves. (Many of these tests have already been described; they involve the functioning of the head, neck, and eyes as well as overall coordination and sensation.)

Positional Testing

This is an examination that includes several different position-changing maneuvers. It is conducted by a physician in the office (or by a technologist in the laboratory tests described later) to try to induce vertigo and nystagmus. The examiner may ask you to wear a pair of special magnifying glasses called Frenzel goggles to make it easier to observe your eyes. The goggles are so thick and magnify so much that you see only a blur. This keeps you from looking at objects in the room that might suppress the eye movements the examiner is seeking. Thus, any eye movements you make are in response to the test, not in response to other visual stimuli.

For this test you may start by sitting, then you will be asked to lie on your back. Your head will be turned quickly to the extreme right and then to the left, holding each position for about twenty seconds. If you experience vertigo, or if rapid movement of the eyes (nystagmus) is noted, the doctor may suspect a proprioceptive disorder in the neck, possibly the result of a whiplash injury or arthritis. This test can also exacerbate a problem within the inner ear, and the above reaction may be indicative of vascular problems.

Hallpike Test

You will also be given the Hallpike test. For this test you may wear the Frenzel goggles and will be seated on the examining table in a position such that when you lie down, your head will be hanging off the edge. The physician will support your head so there is no danger of an accident or trauma. After having your head in this hanging position for up to twenty seconds, you will be brought back to the original sitting position. At all times you will be looking straight ahead (the magnifying glasses keep you from fixating your eyes elsewhere). This will be repeated several times, with your head moved in different directions as well as up and down.

Any nystagmus will be carefully noted by the physician. Depending on the position in which you are placed and the direction of the nystagmus, the findings may be suggestive of some major or minor problems.

After your primary care physician and perhaps one or more specialists have met and examined you, the physician should have a tentative diagnosis or good idea of what is causing your dizziness. At this point, he or she may order blood tests or more technical evaluations.

Subsequent Specialized Tests

Judy, a married 52-year-old advertising manager, had been suffering from a vague sense of dizziness and "fuzzy vision" that was making her uncomfortable and causing problems at work. She had gone to her ophthalmologist and her eyes checked out just fine. She had consulted her primary care physician, who, not finding anything wrong, referred her to a neurologist. The neurologist performed a thorough office examination and, although finding no indication of a problem, suggested she get magnetic resonance imaging (MRI). This high-tech and very expensive test was available at her local hospital. Judy was frightened until the neurologist explained that the reason for the test was to make sure no problem had been missed.

Judy had the MRI, and just as her primary care physician and the neurologist had thought, it proved negative for any medical or structural problems that could have caused her dizziness.

Within several weeks, Judy recovered from her dizziness. The cause? Probably a virus, or possibly some anxiety regarding her concerns over an aging parent who was becoming increasingly dependent upon her.

Why did the neurologist order the MRI? If Judy had consulted an otolaryngologist instead, would she have had a different work-up with the same results?

Unfortunately, the answer may well be yes. Doctors order tests for many reasons. Some do it for legal reasons, hoping to protect themselves against lawsuits. Doctors are never sued for doing too many tests, but they *are* sued for overlooking something, especially if there is a way to investigate it, and the doctor doesn't suggest it. If the patient refuses to take the test, or the insurance company refuses to pay for it, the doctor is still protected against any charge of malpractice.

Dizziness, as you have already discovered, can be a symptom of so many different conditions that there is hardly a test in medicine that some physician will not think is appropriate to order.

Some physicians take a "shotgun" approach, ordering test after test in hopes of finding something. The likelihood that a test will have abnormal results even if the patient is normal increases when more tests are administered. Therefore, according to statistical reasoning, one would expect "something abnormal" (a so-called "false positive" result) to show up eventually if enough tests are administered. Tests don't ever replace a good medical history, yet all too often they are ordered by a physician in lieu of listening carefully to the patient and considering each answer thoroughly. Tests should supplement this process, and some of the new tests replace older unpleasant or invasive ones, also making it possible to avoid exploratory surgery.

Be your own advocate. Be sure that your physician has asked you questions, listened carefully to your answers, and made careful notes. And be sure that the physician tells you why the tests are necessary and what diagnosis is expected to be confirmed or ruled out.

Ear Tests

As you know, the vestibular organs are found in the ears, so it is not surprising that an investigation of dizziness might begin with tests as well as a routine examination of the ears. Since a pathological process involving the ear may cause hearing loss in one or both ears as well as damage to the vestibular system, you may be given or sent elsewhere for an auditory system assessment, an evaluation of your ears and hearing. Much of this consists of the medical history and examination described earlier in this chapter, but it also includes one or more hearing tests known as *audiograms*. A loss of hearing in one or both ears is sometimes indicative of damage to the vestibular system, and audiograms can detect this. Moreover, the tests today are so sophisticated that they can also pick up subtle signs of a tumor or other abnormality within the ear.

AUDIOGRAM. Audiograms, usually performed by audiologists, are conducted in a soundproof booth or room. You are given earphones and a method for signaling when you hear certain sounds. In addition, the audiologist asks you to repeat a number of words. The audiogram consists of two parts: one measures sounds and the other measures the ability to understand speech.

Sounds are measured at several frequencies from low (125 Hz) to high (8,000 Hz) and can indicate if the hearing loss is caused by a problem in the middle ear, the inner ear, or the auditory nerve. Two types of hearing loss that the audiogram is most able to distinguish between are sensorineural and conductive.

Sensorineural hearing loss usually results from an abnormality of the cochlear hair cells or the auditory nerve. Although half of all individuals with this condition were born with it or developed it in childhood, it can occur in adults as well. Taking certain medications or being exposed to loud and continuous noise can lead to sensorineural hearing loss.

Sensorineural losses that are considerably greater in one ear than the other are sometimes associated with an acoustic neuroma, a benign (noncancerous) tumor that develops on the eighth cranial nerve (the nerve essential to the sense of hearing) and grows within the auditory canal. This tumor can cause hearing loss, tinnitus, and sometimes imbalance or an unsteady gait. Other tumors that develop between the brain and ear can have the same effect.

Conductive hearing loss is caused by an error in the transmission of sound from the outside world through the hearing bones, tympanic membrane (eardrum), and cochlea (hearing part of the inner ear).

To evaluate the individual's ability to understand speech, the audiologist either reads or plays a tape of a standardized list of words. The inability to understand and correctly identify a normal number of words suggests that the hearing loss may result from an acoustic neuroma or brain dysfunction.

AUDITORY BRAIN-STEM RESPONSE (ABR). This test, sometimes called brain-stem audio evoked responses (BAER) or auditory evoked response, is based on the principle that sounds evoke a characteristic pattern of brain waves. Any abnormalities in the ear or brain can affect these responses. However, a severe vestibular problem may still produce a normal ABR.

The test measures hearing and is especially useful for detecting an acoustic neuroma. Safe, fairly sensitive, and inexpensive in comparison to some of the newer tests, such as magnetic resonance imaging (MRI) and computed tomography (CT) scans, it is widely used.

If you have an ABR, headphones are placed on your ears and electrodes will be (painlessly) attached with adhesive to the surface of your scalp. You will listen to a series of clicking sounds played quickly through the headphones. The electrodes record your brain waves, and the physician can read the results that appear as a graph on paper. The computer averages the responses of many clicks of sound to arrive at the final result. A delay in nerve conduction between the ear and the brain will occur if the nerve impulses along the nerve pathways related to hearing are impaired. The graph also identifies the location of any problem along the vestibular pathway.

The importance of these ear tests is both to identify problems with hearing and to pinpoint the cause of dizziness. If your hearing is below normal, you may be helped by hearing aids. Various treatments may also eliminate the dizziness. Other ear problems can also be treated, medically or surgically.

ELECTROCOCHLEOGRAPHY. This is an interesting test that is meant to detect the tiny electrical impulses that the ear must generate in order to hear. The impulses are very small and difficult to detect. In order to do so, two tricks are employed. First, the sound stimulus is repeated many times (1,000 may be reasonable). Second, the recording electrode is placed as close as possible to the cochlea.

The test is performed by placing a sound producing device in the same ear as a recording electrode. An electrode that involves insertion of a needle through the eardrum right onto the bone of the cochlea yields the best result. The requirement for a needle is not pleasing to many people, so there are now electrodes that are placed very close to the eardrum. These do not give as good a signal and can be uncomfortable. The electrodes should not cause problems but, as one might expect, there have been a few problems after needle insertion through the eardrum. However, these are very rare.

The difficulty of recording and other factors mean that the electrocochleography test is not as useful as one would like. The results vary frequently when repeated. The accuracy is only fair. There are many research applications for the test, but the main use in clinical medicine is to detect endolymphatic hydrops. It seems that one part of the signal is much larger in people who have Ménière's disease or endolymphatic hydrops. This test is performed quickly and is usually safe, but there are some questions about how much information it really gives.

CALORIC TESTING. The word "caloric" refers to the use of different temperatures. A caloric test can be administered by itself, but it is most commonly a subtest in a battery of tests known as the electronystagmogram. The technique of caloric testing is to place a thermal stimulus into each ear canal separately. Different testing centers employ different techniques. Frequently, both warm and cold stimuli are used. Some centers use water, some use air, and some use both.

During this test, you are asked to stare at a point on the wall or ceiling while the examiner watches your eyes. In some cases, the eye movements will be recorded by electrodes attached to the skin. The caloric stimulus activates the vestibular system, and this activation causes the very particular type of eye movement called nystagmus, the to-and-fro movement of the eyes. The type of nystagmus that occurs during vestibular testing has two phases: the first phase is a slow movement of the eyes in one direction, followed by the second phase, which is a quick, corrective movement in the other direction. The movements are usually left and right in vestibular testing or disease. Up and down nystagmus movements are suggestive of brain dysfunction. The slow movement is dependent upon vestibular function, and it is for this reason that the speed of the eye movement is measured to estimate the amount of the vestibular function that is present. After a wait of five minutes or so, the procedure may be repeated with another temperature or in the other ear.

The caloric test works by causing slight expansion or contraction of the endolymph fluid in the inner ear. This mimics movement of the endolymph, and it appears to the vestibular system that the head is moving. Of course, this information comes from one ear only, since the other ear has not been stimulated. For this reason, caloric testing usually makes the subject feel dizzy if there is sufficient vestibular function present.

The caloric test may be administered in several ways, depending on the examiner's or clinic's choice. Sometimes, the water used is ice-cold; unfortunately, this can be extremely uncomfortable. It can cause a violent whirling vertigo, sometimes nausea. In addition the ice-cold water can cause pain in the ear canal. There are a number of variations of the caloric test. Sometimes warm or cold air, or warm water, is used, which produces less discomfort. Discomfort is also reduced if the ears are irrigated gradually. Occasionally, both ears are stimulated simultaneously.

When the caloric test is administered in the traditional way, without a full ENG (see following page), there are no recording devices attached to the patient, so the velocity (speed) of the eye movements cannot actually be measured. Instead, the length of the eye movement response is timed. The clock is started when nystagmus is noted and stops when it appears to fade away. The traditional test certainly provides some information, but it lacks precision. It is sometimes difficult to determine when the eye movements start or stop, and it is not possible to measure the slow phase or the velocity of the eye movements. (This velocity is the most consistently reliable parameter of vestibular function.) However, the test has merit, and may be done when other more sophisticated equipment is not available. It can also be administered to someone who is homebound or bedridden, avoiding the need to transport the patient elsewhere.

Today, caloric testing has become far more sophisticated, and electrodes may be attached by adhesive to the skin near the eyes. In this way, the examiner gets a more precise reading of the nystagmus. When the test is performed this way, caloric testing is part of electronystagmography, as described on the following page.

Electronystagmography (ENG)

Electronystagmography (ENG) is an umbrella term for a number of tests that assess the relationship between the eyes and the vestibular system, helping to establish whether vertigo is due to a problem within the vestibular system or the central nervous system.

Because we cannot test vestibular sensation directly we use indirect methods to measure the reflex between the ears and the eyes as discussed earlier in this chapter. The vestibular system is stimulated, and then the reactions seen in the eyes are carefully measured. This is more precise than relying on the observation of the examiner or basing a diagnosis on the patient's reports of vertigo or other dizziness.

ENG measures nystagmus, the involuntary movement of the eye with a slow movement to one direction and a quick, corrective movement toward the other side. It is the slower phase that helps analyze vestibular function.

When the vestibular system is stimulated naturally and nystagmus occurs spontaneously, it is either because something different is occurring in the environment or something has gone awry internally. In this laboratory-controlled situation, the vestibular system is purposefully and directly stimulated.

Part of the electronystagmogram evaluation includes a caloric test, as described in the previous section. Electrodes are attached to the patient either on the scalp or near the eyes, and the eye movements are recorded on graph paper to provide a permanent record for analysis and comparison. These tests and their variations (see following) are thus referred to as electronystagmography.

Gaze Test

This test can determine if spontaneous nystagmus is present. You are asked to visually fixate on points, usually lights or dots 20 to 30 degrees to the left, and later to the right, while the machine records your eye movements. If you suffer from a vestibular disorder, you may develop horizontal nystagmus. It is possible to diagnose which ear is affected because the quick phase of the nystagmus is more pronounced when you look *away* from the affected ear and usually decreases as you look *toward* the affected ear.

If your dizziness has been caused by a problem with one ear, the nystagmus may increase or decrease, but it will *always* be in the same direction. This is not true when the cause is a brain lesion, because in that case the direction of nystagmus changes depending upon direction of the gaze. The nystagmus may also be oblique or vertical rather than horizontal, and it can change from minute to minute.

The purpose of the gaze test is to identify any residual nystagmus that may not have been apparent to the examiner without the recording ability of an ENG test. The gaze test is particularly useful if it confirms the findings of the caloric test.

Saccade and Calibration Test

This test is especially useful for accurately measuring the velocity (speed) of the eye movements. You are asked to look at dots or lights that are a known distance apart. In this way, the number of degrees of rotation of the eye can be measured. The test can also be calibrated to accurately measure the velocity. If your vestibular system and brain function are intact, you will look from dot to dot without any back-and-forth eye movements as you try to find each one. Your eyes should move at a speed that falls within a certain range. Eye movements that are abnormally slow or convey that you are searching for the dot indicate a problem. It may be because of poor vision, but if these eye movements follow a particular pattern, they may indicate that the control of eye movement by the brain has become impaired. This is a simple yet very important test for detecting any dysfunction in the brain.

Tracking Test

In this test, you are asked to follow a pendulum as it moves back and forth across your field of vision. While you are doing this, your eye movements are recorded. They should be smooth and trace the path of the moving object accurately. If your eye movements are jerky, this may suggest lack of control or inattention. If the movements follow an abnormal pattern, this might indicate lack of proper control by the brain in its control of the eyes. (Brain pathology is sometimes the cause.) The tracking test measures the pursuit pathway in the brain that works closely with the vestibular system to maintain gaze as the head moves.

Optokinetic Test

Optokinetic eye movements (see chapter 1) are a reflex that causes your eyes to move when the field of vision moves.

For this test, you are looking at a moving visual field. Usually, this is arranged by surrounding you with a large pattern (often stripes) that fills an area as far as you can see. The pattern rotates slowly in front of your eyes. Your eyes pick up the pattern and move so that the speed of the eyes during the slow phase is the same as the speed of rotation.

As your eyes drift too far to the right or left, the fast phase of the reflex occurs, correcting the eye position so that the eyes are able to move again with the pattern observed during the slow phase.

This test may also be done by having you sit in a computer-controlled rotating chair while the visual surrounding pattern remains fixed. By rotating you at a constant but slow speed, the effect is the same as rotating the visual world around you at a constant velocity. In both instances, there is no vestibular stimulation of the inner ear; instead, only the optokinetic reflex will be elicited. This, you will recall, is the reflex that helps keep your eyes on their target when your head moves. In this test, it will seem as if a pattern is moving across your visual field of view.

Because the optokinetic and vestibular systems are very closely related, any peripheral vestibular deficit that causes damage to one ear will produce an abnormal optokinetic response when the visual field is rotated *away* from the affected ear.

This test has been used more in the past than now, for although it provides important information, much of it can be obtained by the other tests discussed in this chapter.

Hallpike and Other Positional Testing

Although the results of the Hallpike test performed with electronystamography are the most accurate, this test can be done competently in an office without ENG machinery.

Like an ENG test, the Hallpike's purpose is to carefully document the eye movement patterns that denote benign positional vertigo (see chapter 4). This is a fairly common disorder in which certain head positions induce spinning sensations for 10 to 20 seconds. The sensation of spinning can be mild or so severe that it places extreme limits on a person's activities and lifestyle.

The Hallpike test can provoke this symptom and provide an objective observation of whether benign positional vertigo is present. If you undergo this test, you will probably be asked to sit up on a table and turn your head either to the left or to the right. After doing this, you will lie down with your head extended over the end of the table, as described earlier in the chapter.

Although the examiner will be looking at you, the electrodes placed on your skin near your eyes will measure the nystagmus both for direction (horizontal or rotary) and velocity. This test, combined with your subjective description of whether you are dizzy in certain positions, helps to determine if you are suffering from true benign positional vertigo or a disease of the brain such as a tumor or some other abnormality.

Other positional tests done with ENG include lying down with your head straight, right, and then left; and lying down with your whole body turned on the right side, then turned on the left side. The test may also be performed with you sitting and turning your head left, then right, and then hanging your head down and extended backward.

Rotary Chair Testing

Rotational testing has been used for many years, even before ENG was available. Today it is fully computerized.

Although perhaps not as useful as ENG, rotary chair testing is based on mathematical analysis that is applied to the vestibular system. By delivering a carefully measured and precise stimulus to you, information can be gathered about your vestibular function.

The most common type of rotational chair testing involves sinusoidal testing. This means that the chair begins to turn back and forth and soon rotates more quickly at a preset level. ENG electrodes and computer-generated analysis help to measure the relationship of the eye positions to the speed of the chair as it moves. In someone with ear damage, there will be less eye movement when the head is rotated toward that ear. This result indicates loss of vestibular function on that side.

Rotary chair testing is usually performed in the dark so that the eyes cannot pick up cues about movement from the environment. The chair is mounted on a very smooth bearing, and if it is rotated at a constant velocity, you really cannot, at a conscious level, determine if you are moving or not. The only clue is the information you get from the vestibular system. This is the information that is computed into the eye movement response.

There are other forms of rotational testing that involve rotation of the head alone, delivering stimuli that are not sinusoidal but are either random or small, pseudorandom movements.

Theoretically, this sounds like a very precise and information-yielding test. However, some people will test "normal" at one speed and not another, and other people may test "normal" a good deal of the time but still have a problem. There are even individuals whose test results indicate problems, yet they feel just fine. Still, the test is a good research tool and can be repeated many times on the same person; it also has few uncontrolled variables. For this reason, it is valuable to compare current functioning with past tests. Rotary chair testing is best used in combination with other tests to make an accurate diagnosis.

Dynamic Platform Posturography

This relatively new and very expensive test is becoming more available. It was devised to examine all aspects of the balance system: the labyrinth (vestibular portion of the inner ear) as well as vision and proprioception (the sensations in the joints and muscles of the legs). The theory behind this test is that if one or more of these sensory modalities are prevented from sending information to the brain, important diagnostic information will be revealed.

To take this test, you stand on a computer-controlled platform while looking inside a three-sided box. This box contains a pattern that provides a strong visual stimulus, perhaps a picture of a city or a mountain scene.

The platform on which you stand can be tilted forward or backward. In some testing centers there may also be a platform that tilts from side to side or turns in some manner. You wear a harness so you don't fall.

The movement of the platform stimulates your feet and ankle-joint sensors to send information to the brain. If you sway or otherwise lose your balance, your examiner will get valuable clues about your proprioceptive system.

Visual input can be easily manipulated. If you look at a visual stimulus, such as a picture, and the platform is stationary, your visual system alone will tell the brain when your head moves. But if the box moves with the sway of your body by sensing the rotation of the body on the platform, the surrounding visual pattern will move exactly as the body moves. The visual information your brain then receives is inaccurate, because your eyes will tell it that your head is not moving.

Still another way to manipulate vision is to remove it altogether. This is easily accomplished by placing a blindfold on you. Your brain "knows" that the visual input is incorrect because it is absent. This means that all information must be obtained from the vestibular system.

By eliminating two of the three variables that govern balance—proprioception and vision—any imbalance is clearly the fault of the vestibular system. This test has not been as successful as doctors initially anticipated. Since people with vestibular disorders compensate for this disorder and since there are many other factors involved in balance, test results can change over time even though the disease has not changed.

Dynamic platform posturography is considered supplemental because it duplicates information available from other tests. It is not widely used because of the expense of buying and installing the equipment. Still, it has its supporters and may someday be standard for testing patients who are difficult to diagnose.

Platform Fistula Test

This test is done on a moving platform that can objectively determine body sway. This test yields information regarding how your middle ear responds to pressure. An abnormal response suggests the possibility of a small opening (*perilymph fistula*) between the middle and inner ear (see chapter 4).

The test is based on the fact that a change in pressure (for example, while you are in a high-rise elevator, nonpressurized airplane, etc.) may cause discomfort but does not cause dizziness because the inner ear is sealed off from the middle ear. However, if you have a fistula, the pressure will stimulate the inner ear.

This test is administered by changing the air pressure in your external ear canal by inserting an earplug while you are sitting or standing on the moving platform.

An abnormal result is reported if body sway occurs simultaneously with the pressure change in the ear. The pressure change is felt as pressure on the skin of the ear canal. However, someone without a fistula who is feeling apprehensive during the test may also sway when experiencing pressure in the ear canal. Thus, this test suggests but can't prove the presence of a fistula.

Other Tests

There are a number of other tests that do not specifically measure vestibular function. These tests are useful in some patients who have particular neurological symptoms or who have had an extensive evaluation without any conclusive findings.

Since some patients with symptoms of dizziness have nonvestibular conditions that are causing them problems, the following tests may have an important role. They are especially appropriate for patients showing symptoms or signs that would make a physician suspect a neurological or other disorder.

TABLE 3.1
WHICH TESTS ARE IMPORTANT?

1 = Unimportant and probably unnecessary.

2 = Some importance, but advisable only if specific symptoms of
a particular illness other than dizziness are present.

3 = Important, and if done for the right reasons, the results may
affect treatment.

4 = Very important and useful in most patients who experience
dizziness.

5 = Extremely important for all patients experiencing dizziness.

Test	Score
Intelligent medical history; physical examination	5
Electronystagmography (ENG)	4
Audiometry (hearing test)	4
Magnetic resonance imaging (MRI)	3
Computed tomography (CT)	3
Auditory brain stem response (ABR)	3
Blood work	3
Rotary chair testing	3
Electrocochleography	3
Electroencephalogram (EEG)	2
Transcranial doppler	2
Holter monitoring	2
Posturography	1
Active head rotation testing	1

ELECTROENCEPHALOGRAM (EEG). Commonly utilized by neurologists to diagnose seizure disorders (epilepsy), an EEG measures electrical activity of various parts of the brain and is also useful in diagnosing brain tumors and other abnormalities. Occasionally, people with vague neurological symptoms have seizure disorders, but generally dizziness is not the only sign of it. A careful and thorough medical history would lead the physician to suspect seizure disorders only if additional symptoms are described by the patient.

The EEG is a noninvasive procedure that takes one or two hours of waking time. If you are having a sleep EEG it will take an extra hour.

For this test, you will be seated or lying down. Nineteen to twenty-one electrodes will be attached to your head. Electrodes can be either stuck to your skin with paste or, using needle electrodes, stuck through your skin. The paste is somewhat messy, but if needles are used, you will experience some pain when they are inserted. The test is otherwise painless. The electrodes pick up electricity from your brain; they do *not* give off any electricity. The electrical activity is passed on to a machine that translates the information into lines on graph paper, much like in electronystagmography.

Flashing lights are sometimes placed in front of your eyes, or you may be asked to hyperventilate (breathe deeply and quickly for a few minutes) to observe changes in the brain waves. If your doctor has ordered a sleep EEG, you will probably be given a mild sedative so that you can sleep during part of the test.

Despite the safety and relatively low cost of this test, it is not especially useful for people whose only discomfort or symptom is dizziness. It should only be done for investigation of dizziness if there are specific reasons for the doctor to suspect that seizures are present.

BODY IMAGING. The term *body imaging* refers to tests involving such techniques as X rays, nuclear scans, and ultrasound, all of which yield pictures of various organs and other parts of the body.

At one time X rays were all that was available to diagnose brain tumors and other serious problems of the brain. Sometimes, special procedures could enhance the usefulness of X rays, such as placing dye in the blood vessels or air into the cavities surrounding the brain, to highlight tumors or other sites of pathology. These methods were often imprecise or inaccurate (as well as unpleasant), and although they are still used in some instances, many have been replaced by newer technology.

Despite great success in visualizing the body in a way that was not even dreamed about years ago, these new tests are often ordered inappropriately. They are expensive, and patients who require injection of a dye into the veins may be uncomfortable. An added danger is that some people are allergic to the dyes used. These tests are appropriate when there is reason to suspect a problem that can't be diagnosed by examination alone or that requires confirmation of certain specific abnormalities.

Whenever a physician suspects a tumor, stroke, multiple sclerosis, or other abnormalities, imaging studies are recommended. The type of study that is ordered depends on the disease suspected.

Generally, an otolaryngologist or neurologist does not perform these tests. Instead, they are carried out in a radiologist's office or in the radiology or nuclear medicine department of a hospital or freestanding facility. All body imaging and interpretation should be done under supervision of a radiologist. Your otolaryngologist or neurologist may also want to review the films as well as see the radiologist's report.

The two types of imaging tests most likely to be performed on someone whose symptoms include dizziness are computed tomography (CT) scans and magnetic resonance imaging (MRI) scans.

Computerized Tomography Scans: This is a type of X ray that takes pictures indicating various depths of the body. Unlike conventional X rays, these scans provide three-dimensional information on body tissues rather than bone structure. Computers and X rays are used to take pictures in cross-sectional "slices," not the flat pictures shown in traditional X rays. The scan or picture appears on a monitor and can also be printed on X ray material.

Unlike regular X rays, the CT scan can actually help determine the size and volume of a tumor. The computer calculates the density of each area, and this density is then re-created on the viewing screen and in photographs. By studying images in sequence, the radiologist builds up a three-dimensional picture of the inner structures, allowing the doctor to estimate with some precision the size, shape, and location of the tumor. The CT scan's sharp images of such details as blood vessels, fluid compartments, and tissue structure within solid organs permit diagnosis that was previously only available through exploratory surgery.

The machinery used for a CT scan is huge. You will lie on a table, which moves into the center of a large ring through which the scan is made. You will hear the sounds of gears and motors as the scanner takes a series of pictures. The table may move you into various positions. This test itself is completely painless.

The CT scan usually makes use of a contrast dye that is injected into your arm prior to the test. If you suffer from allergies to dye, either the test will be done without the dye or you might be given medication to prevent a reaction.

The CT scan is useful for detecting an acoustic neuroma, a common tumor found inside the skull that develops on the vestibular nerve. Vertigo and an unsteady gait are sometimes associated with an acoustic neuroma, although there are usually other associated symptoms such as hearing loss and tinnitus.

Magnetic resonance imaging (MRI) scans: Like the CT scan, MRI produces a three-dimensional, cross-sectional image. It produces visual images even more detailed than those from the CT scan. If you have this test, you will not be exposed to any radiation; instead, radio waves and a magnetic field delineate the tissues. The test is completely safe and painless, and the only complaint patients have is that it is noisy and makes them feel closed in. An injection of a substance that "lights up" tumors may be given.

Because the MRI device is so sensitive, it can detect dead or degenerating cells, obstruction of blood flow, and subtle chemical changes in lesions that may precede gross physical changes. The images provide information about function as well as structure. It can diagnose multiple sclerosis as well as acoustic and other tumors, stroke, and most other diseases or lesions in the brain.

BLOOD TESTS. Almost any disease can cause dizziness. Systemic causes of dizziness are often referred to as metabolic dizziness. The usual symptom of metabolic dizziness is a feeling of imbalance rather than vertigo, faintness, or mild turning. Dizziness is seldom the only symptom of such a disease. Thus, a careful medical history and a good overall general examination should alert a physician to any condition that is also causing dizziness. It is very important that a physician ask you questions and listen carefully to your symptoms.

Blood tests usually are performed to supply information about two types of conditions: occult infections, meaning those infections that are hidden or difficult to observe directly, and general indicators of poor health.

Complete blood count (CBC): The most commonly requested blood test is called the *complete blood count*, known as the CBC. This test measures the number of red and white cells in a given sample of blood. The red blood cells float in the blood, contain hemoglobin, and are responsible for the transport of oxygen to, and removal of carbon dioxide from, the tissues. A reduction in these red blood cells is called *anemia*, which is often a cause of dizziness. The symptoms that usually accompany dizziness from anemia include tiredness or fatigue. Some inactive people may not think of reporting this to their physicians, especially if it doesn't interfere with their lifestyle.

In many infections, the number of white blood cells increases—sometimes slightly, other times dramatically. People with chronic infections may have a white blood cell count that is in the high, but normal range.

Differential: The variety of white blood cells in the blood is also of importance. Many physicians therefore request a test called a differential, which estimates the number of various types of white blood cells in the blood. Certain cell types serve as an indicator of acute infections and viruses.

Erythrocyte sedimentation rate (ESR): This very simple test measures the rate at which red blood cells fall through the fluid of the blood to form a clump at the bottom. The ESR relates to the amount of protein in the blood and will be elevated in infections or inflammatory processes such as arthritis.

Fluorescent treponemal antibody absorption tests (FTA ABS): People who have been infected in the past with syphilis may suffer from dizziness even though they no longer seem to have any other symptoms. Some of these people may never have been aware of their exposure and were never diagnosed. Some may even have a congenital form of syphilis, having been exposed to it prenatally. For these reasons, many physicians include the FTA ABS test, for late-stage (tertiary) syphilis.

THYROID TESTS. Tests of thyroid function are often done in patients who complain of dizziness. An underactive thyroid (hypothyroidism) may cause dizziness in addition to tiredness, cold intolerance, constipation, slowed heart rate, and/or dry skin and hair.

SMA-6. A machine called the SMA-6 measures sodium, potassium, chloride, carbon dioxide (all called *electrolytes),* blood urea nitrogen, and glucose, all important elements for normal functioning. Diabetics whose levels of blood glucose are either elevated or depressed may suffer from dizziness. If a person is not drinking enough liquid, he or she may become dehydrated. Thus, anyone who has already been diagnosed as a diabetic (or who a physician suspects may suffer from diabetes) and who shows symptoms of dizziness will have a blood glucose test to be sure the person's metabolism is in balance.

INNER EAR ANTIGENS AND ANTIBODIES. There are some recently developed special blood tests, not yet available widely, that may identify antibodies directed against the cochlea.

SPINAL TAP. A spinal tap, also known as a *lumbar puncture,* which removes fluid from the spine, reveals information about the brain and spinal cord. It is performed when there is a suspicion of *meningitis,* a serious disease that produces dizziness as a symptom along with a stiff neck, pain, fever, nausea, vomiting, neurological symptoms, or severe headache.

In this test, the doctor (usually a neurologist or neurosurgeon) inserts a needle through the space between the vertebrae (backbone) to remove about one to two teaspoons of spinal fluid for analysis. The test causes uncomfortable pressure, and some people find it briefly painful.

The procedure is often done in a hospital setting, but it can be performed in a clinic or physician's office if provisions can be made for the patient to lie prone for a few hours afterward. This will help avoid a headache. In addition, anyone who has had a spinal tap should be observed for any temporary neurological reactions. Although a spinal tap is not generally risky, there are possible complications. Those who have blood clotting disorders or increased spinal fluid pressure are usually advised not to have the test unless there is no other option available to make a diagnosis.

The test should not be done simply for dizziness unless associated symptoms make it advisable. Since the advent of CT scans and MRI, the use of spinal taps has declined.

ELECTROCARDIOGRAM. An electrocardiogram (EKG or ECG) is the most common test of heart function. During this test, you lie down on your back and electrodes are affixed to your chest, sometimes with an adhesive gel. Electrical impulses from your heart are transmitted to a recording device that produces a graphic reading, and this is later interpreted by the physician. The test is neither uncomfortable nor dangerous.

Dizziness alone, unless it involves feeling faint or fainting, doesn't usually suggest heart disease. However, if you haven't recently had an EKG, it is an appropriate test, although not essential for diagnosing dizziness. The EKG can reveal heartbeat irregularities. Abnormal levels of certain chemicals (calcium, sodium, potassium) in the blood can also be suggested by the EKG.

HOLTER MONITOR. Dizziness is often associated with an irregular heartbeat. The arrhythmia, as it is called, can cause the heart to beat too slow (bradycardia) or too fast (tachycardia). This may cause feelings of faintness. Some people actually do faint.

If a physician suspects that this is the cause of your type of dizziness, it may be suggested that you wear a Holter monitor for a day. This is a battery-operated tape recorder that monitors your heartbeat over a 24-hour period. The tape is then analyzed by a computer for any evidence of arrhythmia.

Although it is a safe and inexpensive technique, many physicians feel that the Holter monitor has been overused in patients whose complaints are minimal or vague. Still others feel that it is useful if the cause of the faintness has not been determined by other means.

Much of the responsibility for a correct diagnosis and treatment of dizziness rests with you—the patient—as well as the physicians you consult.

You need to remember to answer questions asked of you as truthfully and as fully as possible, neither exaggerating nor minimizing the amount of discomfort you feel.

Remember to be a good observer before you consult the physician, so you can describe what makes your symptoms worse, what eases them, and how long they last.

Participate in examinations or tests recommended by the physician, but don't become passive. Ask questions. You should want answers to the following:

- What is the purpose of this test?
- Are there any risks to the test? If so, what are they?
- What, if any, alternatives to this test are there?
- How much will the test cost?
- Does insurance pay for the test?

The medical examination and tests should result in one of the following diagnostic categories:

- Peripheral vestibular disorders involving the labyrinth (inner ear). These include benign positional or paroxysmal vertigo, diseases and trauma to the ear, vestibular neuronitis, perilymph fistula, and Ménière's disease.
- Central vestibular disorders resulting from a disorder in the brain or its connecting nerves. These include brain tumors (benign or malignant), multiple sclerosis, and stroke.
- Systemic disorders originating in nerves or organs outside the head. These include cardiovascular diseases, infectious diseases, blood disorders, connective tissue and arthritic problems, diabetes, and thyroid disease.

Once a diagnosis has been made, you will be able to get the treatment you need to get your life back in balance.

PART II

The Causes
of Dizziness

4

Peripheral Vestibular Disorders

For many people with temporary balance problems, the dysfunction is within the inner ear or its connections to the brain (a peripheral vestibular disorder).

Knowing this may be comforting, for it means you are not likely to have a life-threatening illness. It can be disconcerting, however, because often the precise cause is elusive and treatment may require trial and error.

Physicians with an interest in dizziness are making good progress in diagnosing and treating people, and can usually help you return to comfort and good health. Doctors with little interest in the condition, however, may not give it sufficient attention.

Jack's case is an example. Plagued with frequent bouts of vertigo that had forced him to give up his weekly bridge games and bowling, 68-year-old Jack spent a great deal of his retirement sitting in his easy chair watching TV. Jack's primary care physician, a young man with a busy practice, didn't seem concerned about the vertigo or Jack's health, since Jack appeared fit and his heart and blood pressure were fine. He advised Jack to take a nonprescription medication for motion sickness.

Too bad. A knowledgeable and interested physician would have explored Jack's dizziness more carefully and diagnosed a particular disorder that could be successfully cured, like Ella's.

Benign Paroxysmal Positional Vertigo

For years Ella, a 71-year-old retired beautician, had heard some of her older clients complain that when they put their head back to have their hair shampooed, they would suddenly feel as if the shop were spinning around.

Lately, she had begun to notice some changes in her balance. She no longer bounded up and down the library steps, but instead held on to the rail for fear she might fall. She spent less time ice-skating and skiing because she just didn't feel steady anymore.

Sometimes, when the alarm went off in the morning, Ella turned her head quickly and would develop an extreme sensation of whirling that would subside in about 10 to 30 seconds.

Ella didn't think it was worth reporting to her doctor; she just began to find ways to adjust her life to deal with these occasional bouts of vertigo. She noticed that they often occurred in the morning when she was emptying the dishwasher or making her bed, so she reserved afternoons and evenings for her many activities.

Ella also noticed she didn't remember things as well as in the past. Without a shopping list, she would forget several items on a trip to the supermarket. Sometimes she just couldn't organize her thoughts, so the shopping list would be incomplete. Then, to make matters worse, when she would push the supermarket wagon and simultaneously look at the products that lined the shelves, she became dizzy.

One day, when she was baby-sitting for her eight-month-old grandson and raised her head to get a toy from the hammock above the changing table, she experienced a severe feeling of vertigo accompanied by nausea. Fearful for the baby and herself, she called her doctor for an appointment.

Forty-three-year old Ron had a different experience. He was the supervisor of a warehouse for a large food concern. One busy Wednesday morning he tripped over a package that had fallen off one of the hand trucks and hit his head sharply on a metal shelf. Stunned for a moment, he put his hand to his head and was relieved to find he hadn't cut himself. He felt fine and continued to work the rest of the day.

That Friday, Ron was working at his desk on the balcony when he heard a loud noise. He turned his head sharply to the left to see what was happening and suddenly felt as if he were spinning around in circles. He got up, staggered, felt sick to his stomach, and vomited.

He thought it might be the flu—or possibly a concussion from the other day. Ron went home early and rested, but he felt fine. The next morning, as he was bending down to put on his sneakers, the vertigo came over him again, although not as severe as the previous day. Early Monday, as he rolled over in bed to kiss his wife good morning, he felt as if the whole room were spinning. Ron stayed home and called his doctor.

The Medical Visit

Both Ella and Ron were fortunate enough to have doctors who didn't dismiss these symptoms as inconsequential, and didn't jump to conclusions about diagnosing and treating them.

Instead, their doctors listened carefully to their histories. Although the scenarios were quite different, there was a commonality: They both suffered from vertigo when the direction of their heads were changed with respect to gravity. Neither one had any of the inner ear problems that sometimes accompany dizziness: hearing loss or tinnitus. Their doctors had known each of them and their families for some time, and knew that neither one of them was likely to be suffering from such symptoms because of anxiety.

Their blood pressures were taken (after they lay down and quickly sat up), and each had an electrocardiogram and a general medical checkup, with a special emphasis on neurological function. Nothing unusual turned up, although Ron's doctor suggested he take off a few pounds.

Both Ella's and Ron's physicians were sure that they were suffering from *benign paroxysmal positional vertigo* (BPPV), also called benign positional vertigo (BPV), a syndrome (combination of signs and symptoms rather than a particular disease) that consists of episodes of spinning or vertigo that occur with particular head positions. Commonly, BPPV occurs when one lies on one's back and rolls to one side. Almost immediately, a sensation of whirling or swirling develops that will subside after twenty or thirty seconds. Other head positions, such as looking up or bending down, may also provoke the dizzy episodes.

This dizziness is referred to as "benign" because it is not life-threatening (although it can get you and others into dangerous situations), "paroxysmal" because it occurs suddenly and is brief, and "positional" because it is provoked or caused by exaggerated changes of head position rather than the typical movement that is often thought of as causing dizziness.

BPPV is often associated with head injury, especially in those under 50 years of age. BPPV often occurs in the 50-plus age group as the result of some degeneration in the inner ear, and is sometimes associated with some other peripheral vestibular illness or a central vestibular disorder. Frequently, there is no known cause and it simply occurs spontaneously.

Both of these physicians did a simple test in their offices. They asked Ella and Ron to replicate the experience that had brought on the vertigo. While both patients looked up, looked down, and turned their heads sharply to the right and left, the doctors carefully looked at their eyes to note if they had nystagmus. Sure enough, a rotary nystagmus was present.

The diagnosis of BPPV can usually be made by a primary care physician, just as Ella's and Ron's doctors were able to do. Still, most conscientious family practitioners or internists prefer to recommend further investigation, unless the symptoms promptly clear up and there are no recurrences.

Ella and Ron were referred to otolaryngologists rather than neurologists because their history, symptoms, and examination led their doctors to believe they had problems of the inner ear, and not of the brain.

The otolaryngologists examined Ella and Ron in much the way we have described in chapter 3. Ruling out other inner ear conditions, they both agreed with the referring physicians. Ella and Ron each underwent the Hallpike test (see chapter 3), which was scheduled early in the morning because, like many people with BPPV, they were far more symptomatic in the mornings. Both also had other ENGs, and Ella was given an audiogram. The results of the tests were conclusive. Each suffered from BPPV, and Ron was reassured to learn that this condition usually resolved itself within four months and rarely persisted for more than six months. The otolaryngologist did warn him that recurrences can occur even a year later.

Ella was given similar information but was told that her BPPV probably resulted from age-related deterioration of the vestibular system with the ear. The prognosis for this isn't as good as for someone who has suffered a head trauma, but she was assured that treatment was available.

Symptoms of BPPV

Although Ella's and Ron's stories from onset to diagnosis are quite typical, there are other experiences, too, and anyone who has been diagnosed with BPPV can tell you about his or her own particular case. Usually, the symptoms consist of abrupt-onset vertigo lasting only seconds, although it may seem much longer, and symptoms are often reported to the physician as such. The vertigo is almost always preceded by movement or position change of the head and sometimes the body. It is more likely to occur if the head movement is forward or backward, but looking up or down or even suddenly arising can cause it. Often, it follows head trauma.

Older people, for whom the syndrome is common, usually do not identify head trauma as having preceded the attack. Indeed, many of them say that they have had some mild imbalance or dizziness for some time prior to the attack of vertigo that brings them to the doctor's office. Some people suffer from vertigo that is so severe that they are nauseous and may even vomit. The initial attack of BPPV tends to be far more severe than ensuing ones. However, many patients report that it worsens before it begins to abate.

Children also can suffer from BPPV, although it is not common. Children of any age can develop it, but more often it occurs around the age of four, disappearing by age eight. The child may experience a feeling of spinning and become upset, clinging to the parent, crying, and walking in an uncoordinated manner. This may persist for several minutes and seems to be brought on by head movements. (Adults suffering from BPPV, however, usually do not become uncoordinated or have trouble walking.) Many of these children will develop migraine headaches when they are older, but the reason is not known.

Causes of BPPV

The most common causes are: head injury and degeneration of the vestibular system of the inner ear, infections (particularly those of the upper respiratory or gastrointestinal tract), viruses as well as some systemic diseases, hypertension, and cardiovascular conditions or brain dysfunctions that sometimes coexist with or precede BPPV. Many people who experience an acute attack of a virus that affects their vestibular system (causing vertigo, nausea, and vomiting lasting up to several days) can develop BPPV anywhere from one week to as long as eight years later. BPPV can also be related to other ear problems or diseases. Sometimes there is no known reason why the condition occurs.

One theory behind BPPV is that otoliths (crystals of calcium carbonate that shift their weight according to gravity) fall from the otolith organs (one of the two organs of

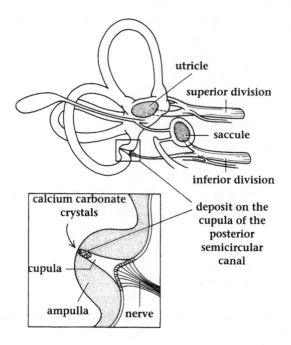

Figure 4.1 Deposit of calcium carbonate crystals that weight the cupula, causing it to move according to gravity.

balance in the inner ear) and become stuck to the cupula (sensory receptor) of the posterior semicircular canal (the other organ of balance) in the inner ear. (See chapter 1 for a full description of anatomy and for illustrations.) Trauma to the head, degeneration, infections, or other problems with the inner ear can cause this movement of the otoliths.

Since the otolith organs sense the direction of gravity, and the semicircular canal senses angular or rotational movements of the head, changes here can upset the balance system. For instance, if the calcium carbonate crystals are stuck in the wrong place, as they are thought to be in people suffering from BPPV, the semicircular canal is stimulated. In certain positions, the canal then reports to the brain that the head is spinning. The brain gets conflicting messages, because other vestibular sensors are communicating that neither the person nor the head is actually spinning. The posterior semicircular canal has been fooled by those little crystals into thinking it is a gravity sensor rather than a rotation sensor, and the canal, now confused, has also confused the brain. Happily, the brain doesn't stay confused for long, and as soon as it has sorted out the situation, everything returns to normal. Moreover, spontaneous recovery probably occurs because the crystals tend to dissolve. But in the meantime, havoc reigns.

In addition to the theory about the semicircular canal, there is a newer one, equally sound, to explain BPPV. It suggests that there is "sludge" or extraneous material in the posterior semicircular canal that moves around and is not attached to the cupula. This matter, which is nothing more than cellular debris, moves when the patient's head moves and causes vertigo by altering the pressure on the cupula. It too dissolves, which results in spontaneous recovery for the patient.

Those physicians who advance this second theory report that they can cure BPPV easily by manipulating the patient into successive positions that tend to reposition the debris. Preliminary reports for this maneuver are good, but most people with BPPV get better with or without treatment.

Diagnosis of BPPV

Diagnosis is made by a careful medical history and physical examination. The definitive diagnosis can be made when the following occurs:

- There is a slight delay between the time the head is moved and the onset of the dizziness.
- The dizziness lasts a short time (10 to 30 seconds).
- Rotational nystagmus is noted by the examining physician or on an electronystagmography (ENG) test when the patient's head is moved to replicate the vertigo he or she has experienced.
- The dizziness is not as severe when retested. One of the hallmarks of BPPV is that with repeated positioning, the amount of the vertigo and nystagmus decreases. This is the result of something called fatigability, meaning quite simply that the reflexes get fatigued and diminish with frequent use, actually lessening the symptoms.

Most people, like Ella and Ron, are greatly relieved to learn that their vertigo is "benign," not due to some life-threatening illness. They are also relieved to learn that in most instances the condition will begin to clear up by itself without any treatment, usually in just a matter of months. In the meantime, many people simply adjust their lifestyle to accommodate it. Naturally, they will be more careful not to move their heads in positions that are likely to precipitate an attack.

As we will discuss in chapter 9, certain exercises are very helpful for BPPV, regardless of cause. The rationale: the brain gets new information so that it can learn or compensate. Medication, even surgery, can resolve recurring and disabling BPPV.

Although BPPV is most often due to problems with the peripheral vestibular system, it can also be the result of pathology in the brain, including acoustic neuroma and other tumors. If the information sent to the brain is correct, but the brain misinterprets and sends incorrect messages to other parts of the body, positional dizziness may occur. For this reason, the physician does at least a brief neurological examination when your complaint is BPPV. Sometimes , a further work-up for neurological problems is warranted, including an MRI.

Vestibular Neuronitis

Vestibular neuronitis (or neuritis, as it is sometimes called) usually strikes people after they have recovered from some kind of viral illness. This form of dizziness has long baffled physicians because it mimics many other conditions.

Cynthia's experience was typical. She had been home from work several days in late February with a flulike virus. She recovered and went back to work, but on Easter Sunday she woke up with a sudden attack of vertigo, followed by nausea and vomiting. She couldn't get up, because every time she tried, the symptoms returned and she vomited. Her daughter was home from college, and by the evening she was understandably alarmed about her mother. Cynthia's doctor was out of town, and the one they reached by phone suggested they go to the hospital emergency room.

The physician who examined her there noted that Cynthia appeared dehydrated from so much vomiting, so they started giving her fluids intravenously. It was also noted that Cynthia had horizontal nystagmus. The doctor wanted to be sure it wasn't a stroke, so Cynthia was admitted to the hospital. During the next two days she underwent numerous neurological examinations and tests, including a CT scan, an MRI, blood tests, and even a spinal tap, all of which proved normal. Tests of vestibular function were scheduled, but by this time Cynthia was beginning to feel better anyway, so she went home. Despite a constant but mild feeling of imbalance, she was able to return to work the following week.

It was several months before Cynthia felt totally steady on her feet. Reassured because nothing serious seemed to be the matter, she didn't consult any other physicians. She never learned what had caused that frightening episode of vertigo.

If Cynthia had seen an otolaryngologist, she undoubtedly would have been diagnosed with vestibular neuronitis. All the criteria were there: a viral infection that appeared to have cleared, followed a few weeks later by sudden vertigo, nausea, and vomiting; no hearing loss; and no neurological signs or other findings.

The cause of vestibular neuronitis is thought to be an inflammation of the vestibular nerve. Cynthia's symptoms disappeared, but a few other people find that the inflammation lies dormant, erupting from time to time over weeks, months, or even years. Generally, the virus does no other harm, but it does cause uncomfortable symptoms.

Bed rest, medication to act against dizziness and vertigo, and antihistamines help relieve the symptoms, but they do not act to eliminate the virus from the body. Antibiotics are of no value, since they are ineffective against viruses. Those people who suffer from chronic imbalance or vertigo often find that rehabilitation (described in chapter 9) can greatly alleviate symptoms, making life far more comfortable.

Labyrinthitis and Other Ear Infections

Labyrinthitis is a term often used imprecisely to describe any problem within the ear that causes vertigo or dizziness.

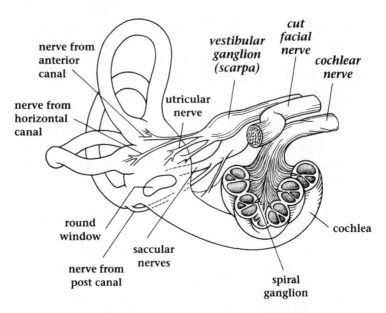

nerve from anterior canal

vestibular ganglion (scarpa)

cut facial nerve

cochlear nerve

nerve from horizontal canal

utricular nerve

round window

saccular nerves

nerve from post canal

spiral ganglion

cochlea

Figure 4.2 Nerve supply to the ear. The hearing (cochlea) and balance (vestibular) parts of the ear give off nerves that combine to form the eighth cranial nerve. The facial nerve (seventh cranial nerve) runs in the same channel in the bone. It controls the muscles of the face.

Viral Labyrinthitis

Most instances of labyrinthitis are viral in origin, and the symptoms may be similar to those of viral neuronitis, but there are some differences. Labyrinthitis, but not neuronitis, can cause hearing loss; labyrinthitis occurs in the inner ear and neuronitis in the nerve. Most people fully recover from both viral labyrinthitis and vestibular neuronitis, although some are plagued with symptoms periodically. Neither responds to antibiotics.

Nonviral Labyrinthitis

True nonviral labyrinthitis is usually associated with a severe bacterial ear infection. It is more serious than viral labyrinthitis. Hospitalization or skilled nursing care at home may be required so a patient can receive antibiotics intravenously. Without treatment, the risk of deafness, brain abscess, and meningitis is high.

Fluid in the middle ear (serous otitis), painful middle ear infection (acute otitis media), and a hole in the eardrum that occasionally exudes pus (chronic otitis media) are the most common types of ear infections. These infections sometimes affect the inner ear indirectly. The dizziness that ensues is usually a constant imbalance, sometimes even a mild vertigo. When this infection or fluid clears up, the discomfort ceases.

Sometimes an infection resides in an area *near* the inner ear. By-products of the bacteria causing the infection can travel to the inner ear, inflaming the hearing apparatus and/or the vestibular system. Nystagmus can usually be seen upon examination. This condition is described as serous labyrinthitis, in which the fluid in the middle ear must be drained and the patient requires antibiotics to prevent permanent damage to hearing and vestibular function. When bacterial infections from the middle ear extend into the structures of the inner ear, it is called acute suppurative labyrinthitis.

All of the above infections can lead to loss of hearing or vestibular function. Some respond to antibiotics more than others. Prompt treatment is essential, especially for acute suppurative labyrinthitis, which causes very intense symptoms and worsens quickly even if treated promptly.

Perilymph Fistula

An abnormal opening between two spaces is called a fistula. A perilymph fistula is an opening between the middle ear and the part of the inner ear that contains the fluid perilymph. This kind of opening occurs spontaneously, permitting fluid from the inner ear to leak out into the middle ear. Fistulas can also be caused by ear disease or injuries that damage bone. Common injuries associated with the condition include a minor or serious fall or blow to the head, a whiplash accident, or strenuous physical activity (especially lifting weights or heavy objects). Childbirth can also cause it. Flying in a nonpressurized plane or scuba diving (barotrauma) is often a factor. A perilymph fistula is difficult to diagnose because it is impossible for a physician to see it upon examination; thus, the patient's history and symptoms are particularly important.

Symptoms

There is much controversy regarding perilymph fistulas. Any combination of dizziness, hearing loss, and headaches is thought by some doctors to be a fistula. Other doctors think fistulas are very uncommon. There are no universally accepted criteria for the definitive diagnosis of perilymph fistula.

1. *Vertigo.* Those physicians who believe that perilymph fistulas are common believe they are present in a considerable proportion of people who suffer from vertigo for which there is no certain cause.
2. *Dizziness of various kinds.*
3. *Ringing or fullness in the ears.*
4. *Hearing loss.* A person may describe a worsening of symptoms because of air pressure changes from air travel, high-speed elevators, and even the weather.
5. *Headaches.*
6. *Coordination and gait problems without any neurological findings.* Exercise or other physical activity may cause a variety of vertigo experiences, as can changes in position.
7. *The presence of nystagmus.*

Overdiagnosis

Even experienced physicians may confuse perilymph fistulas with Ménière's disease, benign paroxysmal positional vertigo, vestibular neuronitis, migraines, or vertigo related to anxiety or other psychological problems. It is therefore quite possible that perilymph fistula is overdiagnosed. In the days before antibiotics, when ear infections were much more frequent, fistulas were more likely to develop. Today, people suffering from the symptoms described should take a conservative approach to treatment. In particular, surgery for a perilymph fistula should not be performed if dizziness is the only symptom.

Diagnostic Tests

In order to determine if you have a perilymph fistula, the physician may conduct a diagnostic test that increases the air pressure in the ear canal. By using an otoscope with a special bulb, or digitally pressing firmly on the little bump of cartilage just in front of the ear canal, the doctor can essentially close the canal. If a fistula exists, the air pressure will be transmitted to the inner ear, causing sudden dizziness. You may also be asked to strain while holding your nose, causing pressure in the middle ear. This may cause the symptoms that are observed by the physician and may be further confirmed by an ENG test. Other tests, such as those described in chapter 3, help the physician to make the diagnosis.

However, the present state of technology and knowledge often does not even allow for a definitive diagnosis during surgery, when direct observation is truly possible. Hopefully, the fistula may be surgically closed and sealed with a graft of fibrous tissue or fat taken from behind the patient's ear.

Treatment

Surgery usually isn't performed—and certainly shouldn't be—unless other methods of treatment have first been attempted. Some physicians believe that surgery should never be the first choice for a perilymph fistula. While surgery can cure or alleviate the vestibular symptoms if the problem is a fistula, it probably will not reverse hearing loss. Moreover, 10 to 20 percent of fistulas are difficult and sometimes impossible to close. The reason for this is unknown. The diagnosis may have been incorrect or the piece of body tissue used to plug the leak may have fallen out. Thus, surgery for perilymph fistula is very controversial.

Since most perilymph fistulas heal by themselves, often the only treatment required is a restriction of activity, usually bed rest with the head elevated. It is usually recommended that a patient avoid any kind of straining. If the dizziness is interfering with regular activities, medications called *vestibular suppressants*, such as meclizine (*Antivert*) are available. Certain mild exercises (see chapter 9) can help the brain learn to compensate. If the symptoms abate, it probably means that either no fistula existed or it has closed spontaneously.

Cholesteatoma

The importance of treating ear infections promptly and thoroughly is illustrated by what happened to one patient. Bob, 45 years old, had been brought up not to run to the doctor with every ache and pain, so he ignored the fluid draining from his ear, even though it had a foul odor and he had trouble hearing. But when he began to feel dizzy and experienced some weakness on the left side of his face, he decided it was time to see his physician.

Bob's diagnosis: He had an abnormal growth of skin tissue in the ear called a *cholesteatoma*.

How does a cholesteatoma develop? Repeated infections of the ear usually precipitate the skin growth, most often in the middle ear, just behind the eardrum. The growth may be in the form of a cyst or pouch, which sheds layers of old skin that are building up inside the ear. If the cholesteatoma is not diagnosed and treated, it will continue to grow and begin to affect the bones of the middle ear, eventually spreading to the brain. If a person continues to ignore it, as Bob did, the symptoms may become severe.

Prior to modern antibiotics, it was not unusual for people to develop a number of complications during or following ear infections. These complications are far less common today, because most people receive and respond to antibiotics. Still, there are people (and not just patients like Bob) who develop a cholesteatoma. Usually it is the result of a partial vacuum developing in the ear because the tube that equalizes pressure is not working properly. Other causes include infections, allergies, or sinus conditions. The eardrum is damaged. Sometimes a pocket may develop because of the negative pressure in the middle ear, so that a sac of skin develops. This sac, if it becomes filled with abnormal skin cells, is called a cholesteatoma.

When a cholesteatoma of the middle ear is found by the examining physician, the recommended treatment is surgical removal. If this is not possible because of other health factors, the ear should be professionally cleaned out and antibiotics and ear drops administered.

Otosclerosis

Some people, as teenagers or older, develop a hardening and new formation of bone in the middle ear. This is called *otosclerosis*, and it can cause hearing loss and ringing in the ears (tinnitus). If it invades the bony capsule of the inner ear, dizziness may also occur. Many ear specialists believe that sodium fluoride may help with this problem.

Trauma to the Ear

One of the reasons physicians take careful histories when people consult them about any kind of dizziness is because its onset can often be traced to some kind of trauma to the ear or head.

A variety of injuries can cause trauma to the vestibular system. A fracture or even a blow to the side of the head where the inner ear is located can affect vestibular function. Constant imbalance and episodes of vertigo may then be precipitated by a mere change in position. Hearing loss may also occur, depending on the location and extent of the injury. That is what happened to Alan.

While waterskiing on vacation, Alan fell on his side and felt his ear hitting the water. It hurt at the time, and by evening he was in excruciating pain. Alan saw a local physician, who told him he had punctured his eardrum. The doctor gave him an antibiotic, suggesting that he see his own physician when he returned home and also to be sure to consult an otolaryngologist. But by the time Alan returned home, his ear had stopped bothering him, and he returned to his usual activities.

When he began to develop problems with dizziness, however, he finally consulted an otolaryngologist. Alan didn't have to tell the doctor about his punctured eardrum—it was evident upon examination. He was also beginning to develop a cholesteatoma, but unlike Bob's, Alan's was still small.

Since Alan's punctured eardrum didn't spontaneously close, he had it repaired in a surgical procedure called a tympanoplasty. A tiny piece of thick tissue taken from behind his ear was carefully placed over the tear. Alan had to keep his ear dry for several weeks, using earplugs when he showered and washed his hair, but he was soon back to normal.

Scuba divers are frequently subjected to an increase in pressure that can injure the inner ear. This may occur during ascent or descent, or at the depth of a dive. During descent, trauma to the middle ear occurs in a condition divers call "middle ear squeeze" (*barotrauma*). It occurs when air fails to enter the middle ear space through the eustachian tube and the diver then experiences hearing loss and dizziness. (Anyone who wants to scuba dive should take lessons from a certified instructor, who will assist him or her in the mechanical precautions necessary to avoid trauma to the ears.)

Someone who has had problems equalizing middle ear pressure should see a physician before diving again. Middle ear barotrauma is not very dangerous, but inner ear barotrauma can seriously damage the inner ear and thus affect hearing and vestibular function. Many instances of perilymph fistulas are linked to such damage.

Ménière's Disease

It all started one day when Grace was rushing from work to pick up her daughter at ballet class. First, there was a loud ringing in her right ear, much worse than the fullness and slight tingling she had experienced a few weeks before. Then, she suddenly felt as if she were spinning around. The dizziness was so bad she had to pull the car over to the side of the road. Then came the nausea and vomiting. In about 10 minutes she felt better and went on to pick up her daughter. Since she remained a bit unsteady for a few days, she assumed she had a virus.

A month later, she had the same experience and this time it lasted longer. Fortunately, she was home and could lie down. After the fourth such episode, Grace decided to consult her family physician, who sent her to an otolaryngologist. Based on her history and examinations, the doctor told Grace he thought she had Ménière's disease. Although the symptoms can vary in intensity and frequency, the classic Ménière's has a distinct pattern of symptoms and progression.

Symptoms

Ménière's disease, first described in 1861 by Prosper Ménière, a French physician, is more a combination of symptoms (syndrome) than it is a disease. They are as follows:

1. *Vertigo.* Repeated episodes of whirling vertigo lasting for an hour or more but less than a full day.
2. *Ringing in the ear.* The vertigo is often accompanied by unpleasant low-pitched ringing, buzzing, or roaring noises in an ear.
3. *Feeling of fullness.* The ringing is sometimes accompanied by or preceded by a feeling of pressure and fullness in the same ear.
4. *Hearing loss.* There is associated sensorineural hearing loss that may fluctuate, worsening in time, while the vertigo may be alleviated.

Anyone can develop Ménière's disease, from children to seniors, but the onset is usually between ages 30 and 50. Many people find their Ménière's to be an inconvenience, but for others it is a debilitating illness. The degree of discomfort is dependent on the frequency, length, and severity of attacks and the extent of hearing loss. It is believed that almost 2.5 million men and women in the United States have been diagnosed with Ménière's.

Diagnosis

Most physicians feel that the only true way to diagnose Ménière's disease is by the symptoms. Vertigo (not imbalance, light-headedness, or other forms of dizziness) must be present before considering this diagnosis. Others believe that some people may suffer from just cochlear or vestibular Ménière's disease. They describe the cochlear form as causing only the hearing symptoms, with progressive loss of hearing. The vestibular type is described as causing spells of vertigo but no hearing loss.

About 75 percent of sufferers have the disease in only one ear; for other patients, both ears may be affected (either initially or later on).

Some people have their attacks in clusters—several attacks within days or even weeks of each other, then none for a long period of time. Others have attacks on a regular basis. Although stress is sometimes thought to be associated with Ménière's, it is not the basic cause of it. Ménière's, however, does cause stress, and it can easily become a vicious circle.

If the otolaryngologist suspects that you have Ménière's disease based on your symptoms, you will be thoroughly examined as described in chapter 3. Nystagmus is usually present during an attack (it is most often the horizontal variety, with the eyes moving away from the involved ear, but sometimes it can be rotary). However, since you are most likely to be examined when you are feeling better, the nystagmus may not be noted. You are likely to have tests of hearing and of your vestibular system, but no test can determine that you do have Ménière's; testing will only rule out other conditions. Vertigo from migraine, perilymph fistula, vestibular neuronitis, BPPV, and other central vestibular disorders and systemic disorders (to be discussed in the next chapters) have similar symptoms.

Causes

As described in chapter 1, two kinds of fluids are found within the inner ear. One of them is endolymph, the other is perilymph. There is general agreement that a cause of Ménière's disease is accumulation of endolymph within the sacs and tubes of the inner ear, creating an expansion of the endolymphatic compartment. This is known as *endolymphatic hydrops*. This overabundance of endolymph produces

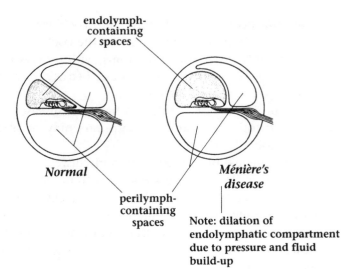

endolymph-
containing
spaces

Normal

perilymph-
containing
spaces

*Ménière's
disease*

Note: dilation of
endolymphatic compartment
due to pressure and fluid
build-up

Figure 4.3 Endolymphatic hydrops. This is the swelling of the middle (endolymph-containing) part of the inner ear, as seen in the cochlea. Some doctors believe that the swollen area bursts, causing severe vertigo.

Figure 4.4 Fluid spaces in the ear. The endolymph-containing space swells in Ménière's disease. It is thought that perilymph leaks out of the inner ear if a fistula occurs.

pressure that interferes with the functioning of the inner ear, thereby affecting both hearing and balance.

What causes this excessive fluid to accumulate? The answer is still unknown. It may be due to overproduction of endolymph or it may be a failure to reabsorb the endolymph. Why does this happen? Here, too, there is no general agreement. In most cases the cause of the endolymphatic hydrops is unknown, but it has been postulated that it may result from an injury to the head, infection, degeneration of the inner ear, or something else that affects the mechanism regulating the inner ear.

There are also differing theories as to just how endolymphatic hydrops causes the symptoms. One theory states that as the endolymphatic hydrops worsens, the endolymphatic compartment swells and eventually reaches a point at which it bursts, much like a balloon. This allows the endolymph and perilymph, which have different chemical compositions, to mix. The perforation where the burst occurred is tiny and repairs itself fairly quickly once the pressure has been equalized. Until the perforation site repairs itself, though, the vertigo attack continues. It is also not clear whether it is the mixing of fluids or the change in pressure that causes the dizziness or the hearing loss.

Another theory states that the endolymphatic compartment doesn't burst, but the swelling (hydrops) in some way causes the vertigo. It is known that the endolymph of the balance part of the ear is connected to the endolymph in the hearing part, so that both functions are affected.

Why is it that hearing loss doesn't always coincide with the development of vertigo in Ménière's patients? One theory is that in some individuals, localized ruptures or damage occur at different times in the balance or hearing part of the inner ear.

In some instances, there are factors that precede the onset of Ménière's and others that are associated with it. People who have had syphilis may develop either Ménière's disease or a similar condition long after being infected. Allergies are reported by some researchers to be a causative factor in Ménière's. Leukemia has also been found to have an effect on the inner ear. Some other researchers have suggested that a number of cases of Ménière's disease are autoimmune in origin. Based on family histories, there is some evidence that there may be a genetic predisposition to developing Ménière's disease.

Course of Illness

In mild cases, even if Ménière's disease is not diagnosed or treated, the course of the illness is not affected. Many people improve spontaneously. Others, however, find that although there is a general improvement in the severity and frequency of the vertigo, the hearing loss does not abate and may even worsen. Because this hearing loss is due to abnormalities of the hair cells within the hearing part of the inner ear or in the auditory nerve, it is considered at this time to be irreversible. Hearing aids can be very helpful in this kind of sensorineural hearing loss.

Although the vertigo may have ceased, elderly people often suffer from hearing loss *and* imbalance, causing major limitations in their daily activities.

Treatment

Many people don't require any treatment at all. They may have consulted a physician after only one or two attacks because they were fearful that they had some serious illness, such as a brain tumor or stroke. For them, reassurance that they don't have any life-threatening illness is enough.

If the attacks or spells are interfering with a patient's normal routine, however, the doctor may make recommendations that will relieve symptoms.

MECLIZINE, ANTIHISTAMINES, AND SEDATIVES. Drugs such as meclizine *(Antivert)*, antihistamines, or even sedatives can reduce the vertigo. They may induce drowsiness, however, and this can impair the brain's ability to learn or compensate. An active, alert brain can do a better job of learning and compensating than one that is under the influence of sedatives. For this reason, these drugs are most useful for those who have only occasional attacks, and it is best to use them only when the person is symptomatic.

DIURETICS. Medications that help the body rid itself of excessive fluid are called diuretics; they are commonly used by people with high blood pressure or heart conditions. These drugs are also effective in treating the endolymphatic hydrops associated with Ménière's disease.

DIET. Salt is known to retain fluid in the body. Thus, a low-salt or salt-free diet can play an important role in reducing the fluid accumulation in the inner ear. This may be the only treatment required for those with mild symptoms of Ménière's.

Some researchers believe that sugar, monosodium glutamate (MSG), caffeine, alcohol, and nicotine should also be eliminated. There is some indication that food allergies increase the symptoms, so it is worthwhile to identify and then avoid any substances that seem to provoke symptoms.

ANTI-INFLAMMATORY MEDICATIONS. There is evidence that Ménière's may be related to a dysfunction of the immune system. Anti-inflammatory drugs that induce the body to stop attacking its own cells can be useful. They range from over-the-counter drugs like Ibuprofen to prescription drugs, such as steroids.

When symptoms are interfering with a person's ability to lead a normal life, and neither medication nor diet helps, surgery may be offered. There are many operations for Ménière's disease, including endolymphatic sac surgery, cutting the vestibular nerve, and destroying the labyrinth.

Note: There are risks, expense, and possible complications with any surgery. The decision to have surgery should never be taken lightly.

At this time, there is no known cure for Ménière's disease. However, there are treatments that can help a sufferer lead a more normal life with a measure of comfort (see chapter 8).

Recurrent Vestibulopathy

There are many people who experience some of the symptoms of Ménière's disease but who don't actually have the full-blown disease. Many otololaryngologists agree that *recurrent vestibulopathy* is an entity unto itself.

The feature that most distinguishes vestibulopathy from Ménière's disease is that it is more likely to improve. If surgery is done for it, it is most likely to be successful, probably because the condition would have gone away on its own.

Some of the ways that doctors can distinguish between recurrent vestibulopathy and Ménière's is that in the former, vertigo spells are shorter—usually no longer than 20 minutes. In Ménière's disease, the spells can last hours, at least at some time in the course of the disease. The reason for this is that it takes that much time for the rupture in the delicate endolymphatic system to heal and for the chemical balance to be restored before the dizziness improves. Another distinction between the two conditions is that usually there may be no hearing loss in recurrent vestibulopathy.

Treatments are similar for both diseases, except that surgery should usually be withheld in cases of recurrent vestibulopathy.

Motion Sickness

Earlier in the book, we discussed how motion sickness can affect everyone under certain circumstances. Some people are so vulnerable they dread each extended car and bus ride and avoid airplanes and boats. Their vestibular systems appear to be especially sensitive to the stimulation that causes the dizziness, nausea, vomiting, and generalized sick feeling of motion sickness. Children over the age of two are more susceptible than adults, but most of them outgrow this vulnerability. There is some evidence that increased exposure to stimulation of the vestibular system provided by car rides helps the child's brain to learn to compensate.

Still, there is no firm agreement as to why some people are more susceptible to motion sickness. One would expect that anyone with BPPV, vestibular neuronitis, or other conditions affecting the vestibular system would also be subject to motion sickness. Yet, this is not so, except during the time a person is experiencing the initial episodes of dizziness. Once a person's brain has learned to compensate, it is no longer necessary to dread a car ride. Furthermore, people who report susceptibility to motion sickness do not necessarily experience dizziness in other settings.

Causes

Research does suggest a genetic predisposition to motion sickness, and it seems to be occasion-specific. Recent scientific experiments were conducted to replicate the setting in which some people experience motion sickness. Results suggested that those people who develop motion sickness secrete increasingly greater amounts of the stress hormones epinephrine (adrenaline) and norepinephrine earlier than do those who don't suffer from the syndrome. Vasopressin, another hormone, will then rise to high levels in the blood of those vulnerable individuals. At that point, contractions in the stomach muscles increase, and you know the rest! Those people who don't suffer motion sickness in the experiments do not show any of these accelerated hormone levels or pulse rates within the stomach. The reason is not known. There are some doctors who believe that increased dietary salt such as that gained by eating salted crackers before or during a trip, will help protect against motion sickness.

Visual input to the brain contributes to motion sickness, but it can occur even with eyes closed or when sleeping.

There is one particular kind of motion sickness—known as pure optokinetic motion sickness—that relies on visual input. As described in chapter 1, the optokinetic system is a reflex that causes the eyes to move when the object moves. Thus, many people suffer intense motion sickness if they are viewing a tilted room, or if the images on a panoramic screen keep moving to allow the viewer a simulated experience of being in a plane or fast-moving vehicle. This kind of motion sickness is triggered by rotating or swaying surroundings, even if the person is perfectly still.

Treatment

Although it may be small comfort while you are actually suffering, motion sickness stops within 24 hours if the stimulation stops. But it might take a few days if the stimuli continues (such as on an ocean cruise), until the brain learns to compensate.

Prevention

There are many preventive measures that you can take if you or family members are subject to motion sickness:

- Before traveling, eat lightly or not at all. Low-fat, nongreasy starchy food may be best. Take along crackers for snacking en route. When on a long trip that requires meal stops, try to eat several small meals rather than a few large ones.
- Help the brain get the same messages from the visual and vestibular system: When flying, request a seat that isn't directly behind a partition—such as the one that divides coach from business or first-class seats. Since this wall moves with the passenger, the visual system is deprived of the information that the plane is moving. Thus, the brain gets two sets of information. The vestibular system says that moving is taking place, but the eyes tell the brain that no movement is occurring. This conflict can increase symptoms of motion sickness.

  Car passengers with a predisposition to motion sickness should sit in the front seat instead of the back. Whether you are in the front or back of the car, look out the front window, watching the curves of the road and not the side window or the seat and floor in front of you. Roll down a window to get fresh air. A cool environment is also helpful, so turn on the air-conditioning even if it's not a hot day.

  On a boat that is rocking, look at the horizon.
- Move your body, particularly your head, as little as possible.

- On buses or trains, face forward. Don't read or even gaze at pictures while moving; this often causes motion sickness. Since children don't usually develop motion sickness until after age two, a car seat facing backward (the safest way for babies) should not cause them to become carsick. Older children may be more comfortable facing forward. A child older than four or five may not require a booster seat for safety but may be more comfortable in one, since it will permit the youngster to look out the front window rather than a side one.
- Keep the mind free of anxiety by either conversing with others or making mental "lists." Anxiety can give rise to the increase of hormones associated with motion sickness.
- Arrange for the driver to fill the car with gas before the passengers (especially children) who are subject to motion sickness enter. The smell of fuel may exacerbate their symptoms.
- Make use of medications that can help reduce or avoid motion sickness. Nonprescription medications such as dimenhydrinate *(Dramamine)* can prevent both vestibular and optokinetic motion sickness. Other drugs are available by prescription. Many people wear a scopolamine patch *(Transderm Scōp)*, prescribed by a physician, when they go on a cruise. The medication is absorbed by the body through a patch on the skin. Some people are bothered by side effects, such as excessive drowsiness and a dry mouth, so try the patch *before* you go on a vacation. From time to time wrist bands and other devices are marketed as cures for motion sickness. Although they sell well, there is no evidence that they actually work.
- Find out about training programs that help people become accustomed to mismatched stimuli. (See chapter 9.)

Height Dizziness

Dizziness associated with heights is clearly not a modern phenomenon. Erasmus Darwin, the grandfather of Charles Darwin, wrote a book entitled *Zoonomia or the Laws of Organic Life* (1794–96) in which he made a number of observations about dizziness that were surprisingly accurate. The book is especially interesting because, at that time, the vestibular system was not yet fully understood by scientists. Regarding dizziness associated with heights, he wrote:

> *Anyone, who stands alone on the top of a high tower, if he has not been accustomed to balance himself by objects placed at such distances and with such inclinations, begins to stagger, and endeavors to recover himself by his muscular feelings. During this time, the apparent motion of objects at a distance below him is very great and the impressions of this apparent motion continue a little time after he has experienced them; and he is persuaded to incline the contrary way to counteract their effects; and either immediately falls, or applying his hands to the building, uses his muscular feeling to preserve his perpendicular attitude, contrary to the erroneous persuasions of his eyes.*

Prevention

If you are seeking a job on a high floor of a skyscraper, or would just like to enjoy the view from the tallest mountaintop or city building you are visiting, don't despair. If you take that job, you *will* become accustomed to the height. If you are contemplating a visit to the top of the Statue of Liberty or the Eiffel Tower, however, you won't have the luxury of time to become acclimated before the tour leader threatens to leave without you. Try the following to prevent vertigo associated with heights:

- Avoid standing without support. Hold on to a railing or lean against a wall.

- If you want to look down, try to find some stationary cues such as the roof of a building that is nearby, or a wall or post that is close by.
- Don't look at moving objects such as clouds or passing airplanes.
- Wait until you are comfortable before looking through binoculars (your own or coin-operated ones available at many sightseeing locations). They restrict your visual field and the magnification sends confusing messages to the brain.
- Don't confuse your vestibular system by putting one foot up on a step near the edge of a railing. Firmly place both feet on the same even level.

You can cope with height dizziness. If these simple instructions don't help, you may be suffering from acrophobia, or fear of heights. Frequently, this phobic reaction to heights follows an experience of intense dizziness. If your acrophobia is linked to other fears or phobias, help is now available (see chapter 9).

It has been suggested that high impact aerobics causes dizziness, but don't give up your sneakers just yet. The physiologic basis for this suggestion is weak, and convincing evidence is lacking. People who exercise or vigorously move their head can expect to feel woozy and experience dizziness. This does not mean that damage has been done to their vestibular system, but rather that the system has been stimulated. The same situation can be seen in muscles or other body systems.

If your muscles ache the day after you do strenuous exercise, that does not imply muscle disease. Movement exercises can be a useful tool in treatment of dizziness disorders just as muscle exercises can be useful for some people with muscle weakness from muscle disease.

5

Central and Vascular Vestibular Disorders

Our complicated balance or vestibular system depends on the integration of two parts: the central nervous system (brain and spinal cord) and the peripheral organs (ears, eyes, muscles, and joints). The vestibular periphery sends information to the brain along the vestibular nerve (eighth cranial nerve). The information first goes to the brain stem, which then sends it to the cerebellum, the part of the brain responsible for coordination. If a problem arises in the periphery, vestibular nerve, brain stem, cerebellum, or somewhere else in the brain, dizziness or a problem with balance and coordination may ensue.

Acoustic Neuroma

For some time, Irene was aware that she was turning the volume up on her television set as well as the receiver of her phone. When Irene, who was in her seventies, went for her annual physical, she told her doctor she had begun to hear ringing in her left ear and had a vague sense of unsteadiness that increased if she turned her head rapidly. Suspecting Ménière's disease, her doctor sent her to an otolaryngologist, who thought the problem was more likely to be an acoustic neuroma. Basic vestibular tests were done in the office (see chapter 3). The ENG test revealed reduced function in the left ear, and audiology tests indicated that Irene had trouble with high tones and with word discrimination. The auditory brain stem response (ABR) suggested that something was impinging on her eighth cranial nerve—the nerve that carries messages between the balance system and the brain. The noninvasive but expensive MRI confirmed the diagnosis of acoustic neuroma.

An acoustic neuroma, as Irene soon learned, is a benign tumor that usually arises on the part of the eighth cranial nerve that carries nerves and blood vessels between the inner ear and the brain. The early symptoms are often just as Irene experienced them, and they can mimic those of Ménière's disease. It is therefore important to get a good evaluation. If the symptoms of acoustic neuroma are ignored for a year or two or longer, the acoustic neuroma can grow enough to severely interfere with hearing and balance. If left unchecked, the neuroma can eventually reach the brain and cause a number of serious neurological problems.

Symptoms differ. Generally, as the tumor grows, it distorts and stretches the nerve, causing it to lose its ability to send clear messages of sound and balance. In certain people, hearing may be most affected; in others, balance will suffer, depending on how the neuroma is growing.

Treatment consists of the surgical removal of the tumor. Balance is almost always restored when the brain learns to compensate for the changes in information it receives. However, hearing loss is usually not restored.

Other Brain Tumors

Other tumors of the brain also can cause dizziness or unsteadiness, along with other significant symptoms. Meningiomas, for instance, are usually benign (noncancerous) tumors that begin in the tissue membranes of the brain and tend to grow large. Gliomas, the most common type of malignant (cancerous) brain tumor, originate within the brain tissue. These and other tumors may have various symptoms, depending on the exact location and type of tumor. They may include seizures, severe or persistent headaches, increasing irritability, personality changes, unusual fatigue or sleeplessness, nausea and vomiting, or difficulties with hearing, vision, speech, taste, smell, and balance.

Sometimes, cancer from another part of the body spreads (metastasizes) to the brain; among the first symptoms of this metastasis may be problems with balance.

Diagnosis of these tumors is made through a variety of tests, including many that were described in chapter 3.

Cerebral Atrophy

As anyone who has ever had increasing difficulty in remembering phone numbers, birthdays or people's names can attest, some brain cells seem to deteriorate as we age.

Often, this brain cell deterioration is vague or slight, and with a little extra time, we remember those numbers and names. Similarly, it seems to take a little longer than it previously did to get back on-balance after getting off a plane or boat.

For some people, however, there are more extreme signs of change in brain cell activity. There may be obvious mental deterioration from Alzheimer's disease. There may be continued problems with balance, chronic dizziness, or bouts of vertigo. *Cerebral atrophy,* the term applied quite generally to the demise of brain cells, can affect balance and equilibrium, and the only treatment may be antidizziness medications.

Still, no matter what your age, you should insist on a careful and thorough medical work-up to see if your dizziness can be halted. No one should passively accept the attitude displayed by a doctor who, upon hearing symptoms, says, "What do you expect at your age?" *Even age-related problems can be treated.*

Disorders of the Blood Supply

Among the conditions that affect the brain stem and cause dizziness are disorders of the blood supply. These are often referred to as vascular disorders. The blood vessels that supply the brain stem also supply the cerebellum and other nearby brain tissues. If for some reason the blood flow is interrupted, dizziness as well as other symptoms may result. Often the one symptom that brings people to the physician is dizziness, because it bothers or alarms them.

Sometimes, arteries twist and develop a temporary kink when you stretch your neck in an unusual way—for instance, to retrieve something from the back of your car. An interruption in the blood flow of the arteries carrying blood away from the heart to the tissues can cause dizziness as well as other symptoms. This kind of dizziness is more commonly a problem for older people who have a narrowing in their vertebrae or spinal column. Some physicians feel that when vertigo occurs by itself in such a situation, it is due to cervical vertigo, which is related to problems with the neck joint. Other physicians describe this as vertebrobasilar ischemia (temporary blockage of the arteries in the back of the neck which feed the brain), a condition that is likely to coexist with other blockages of blood flow. Occasionally, it is difficult to tell where the difficulty arises: in the periphery, the brain, or vestibular nerve. A physician can help sort it out.

Lack of blood flow to the brain can cause far more than dizziness; it can cause *transient ischemic attacks* (mini-strokes) or even stroke.

Transient Ischemic Attacks

One morning, Jim, a 52-year-old salesman, was sitting at his desk writing up orders when he suddenly felt weak on his right side and experienced double vision. Puzzled, and a bit frightened, he got up in order to tell his coworker who was sitting nearby. Jim grabbed at the partition between their desks to keep his balance as everything around him began to whirl, and he could barely speak.

As soon as he sat down on the chair next to the coworker's desk, he began to feel better. But Jim was worried. He remembered that his father, Jim Sr., used to have "spells" like that, and that he suffered a stroke 10 years previously. Jim made an appointment with his physician, which was a wise move. What he had just experienced was a temporary interruption in the blood supply to the brain—a transient ischemic attack (TIA). Most people who have these ministrokes have other signs of atherosclerosis, or hardening of the arteries. These include chest pain (angina) and high blood pressure. Some sufferers may have had diabetes prior to a TIA. But none of this was the case with Jim. He had a healthy cholesterol level and had been taking care of himself by exercising and watching his diet.

Symptoms

Too often, people who suffer from recurrent TIAs ignore them. The symptoms of TIA might include tingling or numbness, usually on one side of the body; vision that is blurred, absent, or double; slurred speech; vertigo and imbalance; and lack of coordination. In a TIA these symptoms clear up quickly; in a stroke they do not.

Even one TIA shouldn't be ignored, because it is an important signal that some cerebrovascular disease exists and that there is potential risk of a stroke. Statistics indicate that about one-third of those who have a TIA will later have a stroke, about one-third will have more TIAs, and another one-third will never have another cerebrovascular symptom. About one-half of those who survive a stroke report a history of TIAs.

If you suffer dizziness with any of these associated symptoms, *you should see your physician.* If you are away from your hometown, or are unable to reach your own physician, go to your nearest hospital. Anyone who has had one of these attacks in the past shouldn't wait for another. Again, see a physician. Don't take a chance that you are among the one-third that will eventually have a stroke.

If your physician has confirmed that you have suffered one or more TIAs, prevention is the key to avoiding further problems. Certain treatments may be recommended to improve the blood supply to the brain. If you have high blood pressure, your doctor will work with you to lower it, through a combination of diet, exercise, and appropriate drugs. You will definitely be told not to smoke, to lose weight if you are overweight, to limit alcohol consumption, to lower your cholesterol if it is high, to keep fat and salt intake to a minimum, and to attend to any other related medical problems, such as diabetes.

Your doctor may make a number of other suggestions based on the examination and tests. Some doctors recommend taking aspirin daily or every other day to reduce the tendency of the blood to clot, thus allowing better flow to the brain. You may be given a blood thinner, a prescription drug that is actually an anticoagulant.

Where there is serious blockage in the neck arteries going to the brain (as confirmed by various tests), surgery may be recommended. The procedure, a carotid endarterectomy, removes the fatty deposits (plaque) from the arteries. This procedure is *not* done to relieve dizziness.

Stroke

When Jim Sr. had his stroke 10 years before his son suffered his first TIA, he was home watching television. It seemed to his wife that he was having another one of his "spells" (TIAs), which he had previously disregarded. But this time his speech suddenly slurred and he appeared dizzy and uncoordinated as he tried to get up. Then he sat back down and seemed all right. Half an hour later, he stood up and said, "I feel funny." His speech turned to gibberish, he grabbed his head as if it were pounding or he were dizzy, and sat down again, his right arm hanging straight down and his right eyelid drooping.

His wife was alarmed. This was different than the other spells, so she immediately called the volunteer ambulance service, which took Jim Sr. to the hospital.

There, it was confirmed that Jim Sr. had suffered a stroke, and he was placed in the intensive care unit for careful observation. Sometimes, symptoms continue to progress or change after the initial ones. This is referred to as a stroke in evolution. When there is no further deterioration, the stroke is considered completed. Jim Sr.'s stroke appeared to be completed when he arrived at the hospital.

Strokes are often referred to by the more technical term, *cerebrovascular accident,* or CVA. There are three chief kinds of stroke:

- Thrombotic stroke, in which a clot forms in an artery, blocking blood flow to the brain. Fatty deposits in the walls of the arteries are usually responsible for narrowing and clogging the vessels. More than half of all strokes are of this type.
- Embolic stroke, in which a clot originates somewhere other than the brain and a piece of it (embolus) breaks off and is carried by the bloodstream to an artery leading to the brain. This can cause an obstruction, cutting off blood supply. This embolism is responsible for about 20 percent of strokes.

- Hemorrhagic stroke, in which a blood vessel in or near the brain breaks and blood spills into or around the brain.

Jim Sr.'s stroke was a thrombotic one, and after a few weeks in the hospital Jim went to a rehabilitation facility. Eventually, he regained almost total use of his right hand and leg, and his speech improved greatly.

Migraine

Jennie, a teenager, remembers the first time she had a migraine headache. She woke one morning with a headache so bad she knew there was no way she could get up and go to school. Her mother was very sympathetic, because she remembered seeing her own sister, Jennie's aunt, go through the same thing.

Jennie, like her aunt, suffered from a classic form of migraine in which the attacks would come on at any time. Usually, sufferers can tell when it is coming because of signs called an aura. Patients describe a distortion of vision in which they see shimmering light. Sometimes they have a ringing or fullness in the ears. Then, within minutes, their headache starts either at the front or back of the head (only on one side), lasting for a day or two. Jennie also developed vertigo and unsteadiness during the attack because there was an interruption of the blood supply to the brain stem. Sometimes Jennie would suffer from vertigo, slurred speech, and tingling around her lips and hands for about a half hour before the headache began. The first time someone experiences this, it can easily be misinterpreted as a TIA, even if the individual is young.

Some people suffer from a condition called *migraine equivalent*. This consists of bouts of vertigo, hearing loss, and tinnitus. However, these persons never (or only occasionally) develop a headache. It can be very difficult to differentiate migraine equivalent from Ménière's disease.

Classification

Doctors consider migraines to be of three types:

1. Common migraine—no aura or warning signs
2. Classic migraine—warning signs apparent
3. Complicated migraine—associated with a number of neurological symptoms that may persist even after the headache has cleared up

Migraine is thought to arise from problems within the small arteries that go to the brain, but is often triggered by certain foods and drugs, hormonal changes, loud noises, and/or stress. There seems to be a genetic predisposition to developing migraine, as exemplified by Jennie and her aunt.

Today there are many new as well as standard treatments available for migraine, and anyone who suffers from the symptoms described above should consult a physician. Some primary care physicians are very familiar with diagnosing and treating migraine; others prefer to send their patients to a neurologist with a special interest in headaches and migraine. Your doctor may recommend one of the new treatments (ergotamine products, a beta-blocker, a calcium channel blocker, an anti-inflammatory medication, or the new injectable medication called sumatriptan [*Imitrex*]) that constricts dilated blood vessels and is reported to eliminate symptoms even after an attack is in progress.

Epilepsy

Epilepsy, also known as a seizure disorder, is not one but rather a group of neurological disorders. It is caused by an uncontrolled electrical discharge from the nerve cells in the cerebral cortex of the brain.

Seizures, as attacks of epilepsy are called, are of various types and severity. The most dramatic type of seizure is called *grand mal.* Although the events will differ in each individual case, there may be rigidity of muscle groups and to-and-fro, uncontrolled movements of the arms or legs. A reduced level of consciousness occurs. There may be biting of the tongue or other dangerous movements.

In some individuals, dizziness may accompany these attacks. In rare instances, it is reported that the only symptom of epilepsy that the person recognizes is true vertigo or mild turning. He or she may experience a small "absence" (lack of awareness), accompanied by repetitive facial movements, but may not be aware of this until an observer calls it to the individual's attention.

One type of epilepsy, called temporal lobe epilepsy or complex partial epilepsy, may have symptoms unlike those usually associated with the disorder. The major sign may be occasional or frequent symptoms much like severe anxiety or a panic attack, in which there are feelings of impending doom as well as shortness of breath, dizziness, light-headedness, unsteadiness or faintness, palpitations, sweating, and a number of other symptoms.

When a patient consults a physician regarding dizziness, it may be difficult to differentiate between dizziness caused by epilepsy and some other cause especially if other symptoms are not reported. When a seizure disorder is suspected, an electroencephalogram (EEG) and a detailed medical history should complete the picture and diagnosis. Epilepsy of this sort, as well as most others, is usually well controlled by antiseizure medications.

Multiple Sclerosis

Only much later did Carin remember the unsteady, "clumsy" attack she had a few years after college. As she said later, "It wasn't just that first attack of whirling dizziness. For days, I had trouble keeping my balance as I went to work, walked my dog, and tried to keep my brand-new apartment reasonably neat.

"I also remember that I thought I should go to an eye doctor, because I was having some trouble with my vision. I hadn't gone in a few years, so I figured maybe I needed glasses. Anyway, it all cleared up before I got around to calling for an appointment, so I forgot about it until something related happened years later."

At that time, Carin was married with two small children, and one day she had a numb, weak feeling in her legs and felt as if she were walking on pillows. She felt dizzy, and she was experiencing blurred vision and trouble coordinating movements. She decided to visit her family doctor, who sent her to a neurologist. He suspected *multiple sclerosis* (MS), a disease of the central nervous system. Based on history, a thorough neurological examination, and an MRI, the diagnosis was definitively made.

Approximately 30 percent of afflicted people experience vertigo as a symptom of MS. Other symptoms include:

- Weakness, numbness, or even paralysis in one or both arms or legs
- Blurred vision or transient loss of vision in one eye
- Pain and impaired vision during movement (usually in one eye)
- Imbalance, tremor, lack of coordination, or unsteadiness while walking
- Involuntary, spontaneous eye movements (nystagmus) of any type, including horizontal, direction-changing, or vertical

The symptoms of MS occur because of damage to the protective sheath, or myelin, that insulates the nerve fibers. The cause is not known, although some sort of virus is suspected. There seems to be some genetic predisposition to developing MS, and it is believed that it may actually begin before the midteens, even if it doesn't produce symptoms at that time. In general, symptoms come and go, and there are periods with no symptoms until the disease progresses. MS is more prevalent in cold climates than in warm ones, and more women than men develop it. Research has produced many new treatments that enable people with MS to lead longer and more normal lives.

Other Central Vestibular Disorders

Tumors or other disorders of the brain, nerves, or arteries leading to the brain can cause numerous symptoms, of which dizziness is just one. For this reason, dizziness or vertigo by itself is usually not cause for great alarm. It is often reassuring to learn it is not the only symptom of a stroke, a brain tumor, or some other neurological disorder. It is, however, the symptom that most often brings someone to the physician for an assessment.

6

Systemic Disorders

Many times, dizziness is just one of many symptoms of a general, systemwide disease or toxic reaction to a substance. It is necessary in these cases to treat the underlying disease in order to adequately treat the dizziness.

Cardiovascular Diseases

Greg, 66, was enjoying Father's Day at his daughter's home when he suddenly became light-headed and felt slightly dizzy. The next thing he knew, he found himself stretched out on the couch with his worried family standing over him.

"It must have been the excitement with all the children and the heat," said Greg after realizing he had fainted. But Greg's family insisted that he call his doctor on Monday morning.

When Greg saw his doctor, he underwent a thorough examination and some tests; then the doctor sent him to a cardiologist.

Arrhythmia

Greg's diagnosis: He was suffering from arrhythmia, a disorder of his heart rate and rhythm. In arrhythmia, the heart rate is either too fast or too slow, or has an irregular rhythm. Some people suffer from chest discomfort, shortness of breath, palpitations, spells of light-headedness, or even fainting, which was Greg's first warning. Other heart problems can also cause these symptoms.

The heart is a hollow, fist-sized mass of muscle that normally beats about 70 times a minute as it coordinates nerve impulses and muscular contractions. The part of the heart responsible for sending blood into the arteries is the left side; the right side receives the blood from the veins to the heart for recirculation. Both sides of the heart beat at the same time but independently of each other.

This system isn't foolproof, and abnormalities of rhythm can cause dizziness and imbalance.

Generally, arrhythmia is related to one of a number of conditions:

- *Ectopic atrial heartbeat:* a rather harmless condition that is just a variation of an otherwise normal pulse. It feels much like a "missed heartbeat." Use of tobacco, alcohol, or caffeine can trigger the attacks. This usually does not cause dizziness.
- *Atrial fibrillation and flutter:* a mild or sometimes serious condition in which there are rapid contractions of the upper chambers of the heart, or atria. This can cause dizziness, fainting spells, and other symptoms. The condition may occur without heart disease; it may be related to heart attack, structural problems, past illness, or a thyroid condition; or it may have no apparent cause at all.
- *Paroxysmal atrial tachycardia:* a condition in which the atria beat about 180 times a minute, two to three times the normal rate. It makes you feel as though your heart is racing, but it is not a life-threatening problem.

Nevertheless, repeated attacks are sometimes related to future heart failure. This is usually not identified with forms of dizziness, although anxiety may cause it.

* *Ventricular tachycardia and fibrillation:* a serious condition in which the lower chambers of the heart, the ventricles, contract too rapidly without being coordinated with the upper heart chambers. Pumping of the blood may be severely diminished. If prolonged, this condition can lead to loss of consciousness and death.

If your primary care physician suspects that a heart arrhythmia is the cause of your light-headedness or fainting, you, like Greg, will probably be referred to a cardiologist.

At the cardiologist's office you will be examined thoroughly with a stethoscope and have your blood pressure taken while you are in several positions. You will also have an EKG and possibly other tests. In chapter 3, we discussed the ways that a blood pressure problem or medications to control it can cause dizziness. High or low blood pressure, or a differential pressure in each arm or in arms and legs, may suggest the source of the problem.

The physician will probably focus on those problems that are most likely to cause dizziness, including arrhythmias and problems with the aorta or any of the valves.

A number of medications can successfully treat arrhythmia. Sometimes, artificial cardiac pacemakers to regulate the heartbeat may be surgically implanted for temporary or permanent use.

Valve Problems

Two particular valve problems can cause dizziness: narrowing within the aorta (the main artery coming from the heart) or a malfunction of the aortic valve. Some people have congenital disorders (they are born with them), and others develop them later. Cardiovascular problems frequently occur when the aortic valve no longer shuts tightly.

Surgery to remove a narrowing in an aorta or to replace an aortic valve, as well as other procedures to correct congenital or acquired defects, have become almost routine.

People who suffer from mitral valve prolapse can occasionally suffer from dizziness as well as heart palpitations, although this condition is more often symptom-free. The mitral valve, located on the left side of the heart, links the upper chamber (atrium) to the lower chamber (ventricle). The valve consists of two leaflets controlling movement of blood between the two chambers. If one or both of the leaflets balloon out (prolapse), this causes extra clicking sounds that can be heard with a stethoscope. The diagnosis can be confirmed by an echocardiogram. Although generally harmless, mitral valve prolapse puts people at risk of developing an infection in the heart. The risk is especially great following dental work (including cleaning and tooth extraction) and certain surgical procedures (tonsillectomy, dilation and curettage [D & C], and others). For this reason, antibiotics are recommended prior to and immediately following such procedures.

Tests

You will probably have a chest X ray, basic electrocardiogram, and some of the following tests:

- *An echocardiagram* (a sonogram of your heart)
- *A stress test.* This is an electrocardiogram performed while you are on a treadmill. Sometimes you are injected with thallium, a radioactive chemical that helps visualize any cardiovascular problems.
- *A Holter monitor,* in which electrodes are attached to your chest and linked to a recording device. The test measures your heartbeat over a 24-hour period or more. You go about your usual activities during this period, then return to the physician with your "record." This, along with a diary-like history that you

will present, is especially useful for measuring heart arrhythmias, a frequent cause of dizziness.

- *Ultrasound or sonograms of the aorta,* or other arteries that may be blocked.

If your dizziness is a symptom of some underlying cardiovascular condition, in all likelihood there is appropriate treatment available.

Bacterial and Viral Diseases

Dizziness is a common symptom in vestibular neuronitis, which is caused by a virus, as well as in viral and bacterial labyrinthitis (see chapter 4).

Many common illnesses such as influenza or flulike illnesses can cause dizziness. When fever accompanies the illness, some people become light-headed or develop vertigo. Generally, the dizziness clears up as the illness gets better. People may be more inconvenienced or alarmed by the symptom of dizziness than they are by other accompanying symptoms. However, it is those other symptoms that offer important clues to the nature of the illness.

Any dizziness that continues unabated or that constantly recurs should be brought to the attention of a physician. Based on your medical history and the initial examination, your doctor will begin to consider some possibilities and eliminate others.

Following are some viral and infectious illnesses that are often accompanied by dizziness, because they have affected the peripheral or central vestibular system:

Herpes Zoster

Herpes is a viral infection that can range from mild to severe. It sometimes produces small, painful, fluid-filled blisters on the skin or along the route of sensory nerves. It can also cause a disease known as shingles. Herpes zoster oticus affects the external ear and may travel along a facial nerve. It can cause hearing loss and vertigo. Medication is available today that attacks the herpes virus, so it is usually not the debilitating illness it often was in the past.

Tuberculosis

A chronic bacterial infection that usually affects the lungs but can also spread throughout the body, TB has been reported to occasionally lodge in the labyrinth, causing vestibular symptoms. Drugs used in the past to treat TB, particularly streptomycin, also affected the eighth cranial nerve.

Syphilis

Syphilis is spread by a spiral-shaped bacterium during sexual contact. It can also be passed on by a mother to her unborn child, causing congenital syphilis. Syphilis responds well to penicillin and other drugs, but if it is not sufficiently treated, it can develop into its third stage within 3 to 15 or more years. At that time, it may involve almost any part of the body, including the nervous system. For this reason, when dizziness and other balance problems are present without clear explanation, physicians often order a blood test to determine if the dizziness is due to syphilis.

Meningitis

This is an acute viral or bacterial infection of the membranes covering the brain and spinal cord. It may follow a sore throat, a cold, or some other illness, or may begin spontaneously. Symptoms are usually acute, and may include fever, headache, confusion, drowsiness, and stiff neck, as well as dizziness. This can be a life-threatening illness, and medical attention should not be delayed.

Encephalitis

This is an acute inflammatory disease of the brain that often results from a direct attack by a virus although it may be a complication of another infection (chicken pox, influenza, measles, herpes, or hepatitis). Symptoms include headache, neck pain, fever, nausea, and vomiting. Sometimes, prior to these acute symptoms, other neurological disturbances of a more vague nature may occur, including dizziness. This, too, is a life-threatening illness that requires immediate medical attention.

Lyme Disease

An infectious disease that can affect many parts of the body, Lyme disease is caused by a microorganism and is transmitted by a bite from a pinhead-sized tick. Anyone can get it, and a pregnant woman can pass it on to her unborn child. If you don't know you were bitten by a tick, and don't develop the typical circular rash surrounding a pale area where the tick had attached itself, the disease may go unnoticed. If undiagnosed and untreated, Lyme disease can progress, causing muscle soreness, joint pain, swelling, and general malaise. The heart, brain, and nerves can also be affected. Neurological symptoms can include dizziness, and this may well be a predominant symptom. Diagnosis is made by blood tests, symptoms, and a medical history, but there are often conflicting test reports and sometimes disagreement among physicians about what the patient's illness really is. Once there is a final diagnosis of Lyme disease, treatment is with antibiotics.

Connective Tissue and Arthritic Problems

Arthritis is an inflammatory condition of the joints, and osteoarthritis, the common form in which one or many joints undergo degenerative changes, can cause problems with balance. The inability to move your head due to cervical arthritis or problems with the feet and ankles can interfere with the vestibular system's ability to gather information that it needs to keep you on-balance. Arthritis can also occur in the vestibular system itself.

So-called connective tissue diseases also produce arthritic-like symptoms. These diseases result from inflammation of collagen, the fibrous protein found in the skin, bone, ligaments, and cartilage, including the ear. This inflammation can cause dizziness.

One of the connective tissue diseases that affects many people is systemic lupus erythematosus (SLE, also known as lupus), a chronic disease that affects joints, skin, and major organs. Because lupus involves the joints, messages to the vestibular system can go awry. Other illnesses that affect the joints are, like lupus, thought to be the result of a malfunction of the body's own defense system and are called autoimmune diseases.

Blood Disorders

A number of blood diseases cause dizziness. These include:

Anemia

When the iron-rich hemoglobin contained in the red blood cells is diminished, anemia can result. There are different types of anemia, depending on what part of the red blood cells is affected. Moreover, anemia may be caused by many factors including deficiencies in iron, vitamin B_{12} (causing pernicious anemia) or another B vitamin, folic acid or folate (causing folic acid anemia), which is needed for the production of red blood cells.

Symptoms are often subtle, and sometimes dizziness is the first one noticed. Other symptoms may include fatigue, pallor, low appetite, weight loss, and problems with balance or gait.

Sickle-Cell Anemia

In this form of anemia, the red blood cells change shape and cause painful attacks, making the body vulnerable to infections. (This is an inherited disorder that strikes persons of African, Southwest Asian, and Mediterranean descent.)

Leukemia

This is cancer of the blood-forming tissues, including the bone marrow and lymph system. Leukemia causes an excess of abnormal white blood cells, the cells that ordinarily fight infections. A high concentration of white blood cells can interfere with the functioning of vital organs. The production of red blood cells, which carry oxygen to the tissues, and platelets, which aid in preventing bleeding and blood clotting, is also impaired. Bleeding or difficulty fighting off infections may result.

Although there are many symptoms, including fatigue, fever, bruising of skin, swollen glands, and weight loss, many people report significant imbalance and light-headedness.

Polycythemia

This occurs when the bone marrow produces too many red blood cells. The high concentration of both red and white blood cells can interfere with the flow of blood through blood vessels. Quite logically, this can lead to a sense of fullness in the head, light-headedness, and dizziness. Other symptoms include weakness, itching, and redness of face and hands.

Diabetes

Diabetes (or diabetes mellitus, the formal term) is a condition in which the body fails to satisfactorily utilize sugar, starches, and other foods as energy. According to the American Diabetes Association in 1994, it is estimated that 14 million Americans have been diagnosed with diabetes and that about half of them are unaware of it.

There is a definite genetic predisposition to the disease. People who are overweight or elderly are more likely to develop diabetes than others. Fortunately, for most of them the disease can be controlled with diet and medication. There is a more severe form of diabetes that occurs in younger persons, which requires insulin injection.

The chief signs and symptoms are increased thirst, unexplained weight loss and/or increased appetite, and increased amount and frequency of urination. Some diabetics may also experience weakness, fatigue, nausea, pain or cramps in legs, frequent or persistent skin or bladder infections, itching, or blurred vision. Doctors routinely check for diabetes, but if you are experiencing any of the above symptoms, you should consult a physician. A primary care doctor can easily and quickly determine the concentrations of glucose in your blood and urine.

If you are diabetic, one of the noticeable symptoms may be dizziness.

Art, 40, loves sweets, especially sodas. Little by little, Art put on a lot of weight, and when he found he needed to urinate more than ever, he simply attributed it to all the sodas he was drinking.

Art began to feel light-headed and a bit off-balance sometimes, especially when he had to climb the subway stairs to get to work. And he was losing weight, with no effort on his part. Still, he ignored it. In fact, he didn't see a doctor until his eyeglasses broke and he went to check his prescription. The ophthalmologist noted the deterioration of the blood vessels of the retina (a long-term complication of diabetes) and suggested he see a primary care doctor. By the time Art saw the physician, he was complaining of unsteadiness on his feet. By then, his diabetes was so out of control that he had to be admitted to a hospital.

Even diabetics whose disease is normally under control may sometimes suffer from dizziness if the concentration of glucose becomes too low. Hypoglycemia, as it is called, can occur if the dose of insulin or oral medication is too high, a meal is missed, or there is more activity than usual. Many diabetics have blood glucose meters at home and have learned to monitor their levels efficiently, so this doesn't happen as much today as it did in the past. Still, diabetics and their family members, friends, and coworkers should know that light-headedness, dizziness, or balance problems can be symptoms of a decrease in glucose. If not corrected this can lead to more severe symptoms that can culminate in loss of consciousness.

Chronic Kidney Disease

People who suffer from advanced kidney disease and receive dialysis may suffer some peripheral neuropathy, resulting in severe unsteadiness. Certain antibiotics normally cleared by the kidneys can also damage the vestibular labyrinth of the inner ear, causing various forms of dizziness, including vertigo.

Thyroid Disorders

The thyroid gland, located at the base of the neck, wraps around the windpipe. An overactive thyroid (hyperthyroidism) produces too much of the thyroid hormone. This causes a number of symptoms, including a tremor of the hands, rapid heartbeat (arrhythmia), and difficulty in sleeping. Rapid heartbeat, as described earlier, can cause dizziness.

When too little thyroid hormone is produced (hypothyroidism), there are other symptoms. These include a slowdown of physical and mental functions, including heart rate. This decreased function has been associated with some neurological disorders such as lack of coordination and sensorineural hearing loss.

Allergies

You can develop allergies at any time in your life, experiencing unpleasant reactions to various pollens, foods, or chemicals to which you have been exposed. Strange as it seems, some people's only allergic reaction is that they become dizzy.

A good way to find out for yourself if your dizziness might be related to allergies is to keep a diary. Are you worse during certain times of the year? Do you feel better if you are able to stay in an air-conditioned environment? Do you notice that certain foods or perfumes seem to cause the dizziness? If so, do what you can to avoid these allergens and discuss any possible causes with your physician. Nonprescription or prescription antihistamines may solve your problem.

Temporomandibular Joint Disorders (TMJ)

Temporomandibular joint disorders, often abbreviated as TMJ, are problems that affect the jaw joint and its muscles. These disorders are sometimes difficult to diagnose because the symptoms can be so varied. Most often, the person experiences pain in the jaw or head. Headaches, neckaches, toothaches, dizziness, ringing or stuffiness in the ears, clicking of the jaw when opened, and problems opening and closing the mouth can all be symptoms of TMJ. Many dentists have made a specialty of treating TMJ, using a variety of techniques. Treatment usually consists of one or more of the following: cold and heat therapy; limiting the patient's jaw movement; pain-relieving medications; anti-inflammatory drugs; special splints or bite plates worn in the mouth to keep the jaws from closing completely; physical therapy; and in some severe cases that don't respond to these treatments, surgery. If TMJ causes dizziness (and some health professionals doubt this) it is a feeling of imbalance rather than vertigo. This dizziness may be anxiety-related in some but certainly not all TMJ sufferers.

Medications and Other Substances

The expression "If something is good, more is better" is certainly not true of medications. Many drugs that serve people well can, in excess, cause toxic reactions that result in dizziness or more serious conditions. Other medications, even when used correctly, can cause dizziness in some people at certain times. In most instances, side effects usually disappear when the medications are discontinued.

Aspirin is a drug that almost everyone has taken in moderate doses. But accidental or intentional overdose is fairly common, and some people suffer adverse effects from only a few aspirin. Symptoms include tinnitus, imbalance, central nervous system disturbances, and gastrointestinal or breathing problems. Aspirin is derived from salicylic acid, as are some other medications, especially those used for anti-inflammatory purposes.

Streptomycin, an excellent antibiotic, can cause damage to the vestibular system if taken in excessive quantities. When the drug was first introduced and used intravenously for long periods of time, especially for tuberculosis, some people suffered irreversible damage. This is unlikely to occur now that physicians are aware of the drug's potential hazards.

People who suffer from seizure disorders are usually given medications called anticonvulsants. These can sometimes cause dizziness or light-headedness, especially if the dose is more than an individual can tolerate. For this reason, patients are told to report symptoms, and blood levels of these drugs are checked on a regular basis to be certain that the dose is appropriate.

People with high blood pressure (hypertension) often take medications that bring the pressure down but can cause light-headedness. This symptom may occur when getting out of bed in the morning, because blood pressure may drop with any change in the body's position. The drugs themselves may even cause dizziness. If the latter case is true, the doctor can usually find a substitute medication or adjust the dosage.

Antihistamines, used for allergies, often cause dizziness. Paradoxically, antihistamines are also used to prevent motion sickness, nausea, and vomiting.

Dizziness is a side effect of a number of drugs used for anxiety and depression. Symptoms can be alleviated by an adjustment of the dosage.

Many people take quinine either to treat or prevent malaria and some take it to prevent nocturnal leg cramps. In some people, in specific doses, quinine can cause dizziness.

Standard drugs for severe pain have historically caused imbalance and dizziness. Many new medications are available today, however, that do not cause dizziness. Other drugs, including recreational drugs, can affect the vestibular system either temporarily or permanently. When exploring your own symptoms of dizziness, be sure to tell your doctor about any drug you are taking.

People who are being treated for cancer are often given very powerful anticancer drugs, known as chemotherapy. Treatment often consists of a combination of different chemical substances that work internally and invisibly throughout the body. A number of the drugs cause nausea, hearing loss, tinnitus, dulling, tingling and loss of sensation in the arms or legs, low blood sugar, and anemia, all of which can be accompanied by dizziness. These are in addition to numerous other side effects, including cardiovascular problems and hair loss.

Mixing almost any medication with alcohol can produce adverse results; dizziness may be one of them. Always read package inserts on drugs, and ask your doctor about drug interactions and potential side effects. Your pharmacist is also a good source of information.

Other Substances

Caffeine in coffee, tea, sodas, chocolate, and some nonprescription medications that alleviate pain, curb appetite, or keep one awake can cause dizziness. Alcohol has long been recognized as causing problems with balance. Someone who has consumed too much alcohol will often stagger and feel dizzy. Alcoholism, whether chronic or acute, can cause loss of nerve cells and consequently dizziness. A vitamin B deficiency, often caused by alcoholism, is also associated with inflammation and degeneration of the peripheral nerves (neuropathy), which result in unsteadiness. However, vitamin deficiency and neuropathy may occur separately.

People who smoke excessively can develop nicotine poisoning, a condition that results in numbness in fingers, dizziness, or other related symptoms.

Other Factors

Malnutrition can cause dizziness. Nutritional deficiencies, especially vitamin B deficiencies, can be caused by alcoholism, poor eating habits, or malabsorption of essential nutrients.

Conversely, megadoses of vitamin A and niacin can cause vertigo and headaches.

Sunstroke can also cause dizziness. In severe cases, body temperature can rise to a dangerously high level. If you have been out in the sun, or the weather is excessively hot and you are feeling dizzy, take first-aid measures. Lie down, try to cool off, apply an ice pack or crushed ice to your face and head, or get into a cold shower.

Pollution

People who are exposed to certain industrial solvents may experience vertigo and nausea. This usually develops gradually over several years, and can affect the central nervous system.

It has also been reported that people working in certain commercial buildings suffer from "sick building syndromes." Symptoms include irritation of eyes, nose, throat, and skin; respiratory ailments; headaches; dizziness; and confusion. These symptoms usually diminish when people leave these buildings. A number of factors have been implicated in sick building syndrome including ventilation, light intensity, carpeting, crowding, the presence of cigarette smoke, and volatile organic compounds. There are many physicians who doubt that sick building syndrome has an organic cause in all cases.

> One of the reasons so many people suffer from dizziness is because it can be a symptom of so many diseases and conditions. That is why it is very important for a patient to give, and the doctor to obtain, a careful medical history that includes everything from daily intake of vitamins to previous allergic attacks. Even if you think an odd situation or condition could have no relationship to your current dizzy spells, be sure to discuss it with your doctor.

Dizziness and Anxiety

After a doctor has done all the appropriate tests and found no convincing physical explanation for your dizziness, the physician might suggest that the cause is psychological. This does not mean it doesn't exist, but it might be a symptom of another underlying problem.

Anxiety

There are a number of physical symptoms associated with anxiety. Anxious people often complain that they have trouble breathing, when in fact they are breathing faster and more than necessary. This hyperventilation causes a lack of carbon dioxide in the blood that produces lightheadedness, numbness in the fingers or toes, and faintness.

145

Other symptoms of anxiety include:

- shortness of breath
- dizziness
- unsteady feelings or faintness
- palpitations, as if the heart is racing
- trembling or shaking
- sweating, hot flashes, or chills
- choking
- upset stomach
- numbness or tingling sensations
- chest pain or discomfort
- trouble breathing
- lump in throat

Panic Disorders or Attacks

Panic attacks come on suddenly, usually with no warning. Such attacks are unpredictable and terrifying in themselves because they are so intense and because they often resemble heart attacks. Panic attacks are accompanied by at least four of the symptoms listed above. They may come on quickly and concurrently and be perceived as dizziness and faintness. Actual fainting might occur.

Phobias

Those who experience terror, dread, or panic at the thought, sight, or confrontation with an object, situation, or activity they fear are described as having phobias. Some common phobias are social phobia, simple phobia, agoraphobia, and acrophobia.

Social phobia is the fear of situations in which a person will be watched by others and will do something that will prove humiliating. A common social phobia involves public speaking, but the term includes almost any situation involving other people.

Simple phobia is a fear of specific objects or situations. Fear of dogs, cats, flying, closed spaces (claustrophobia), or seeing blood are fairly common simple phobias.

Agoraphobia is a fear of being alone in a public place with no easy exit. People who suffer from this try to avoid traveling by public transportation, walking or standing in a crowd, and even going out of the house alone. When faced with such a situation, they often experience dizziness.

Acrophobia is a fear of heights, and it may begin because of actual physical dizziness. However, many people suffer from acrophobia as a phobic manifestation of anxiety.

Phobic Vertigo

Some physicians who treat dizzy patients have also described a condition they call phobic vertigo. People who suffer from this have a frightening feeling of dizziness and think they are about to fall, whether they are sitting, standing, or walking. These symptoms may arise spontaneously or in certain situations, but usually the patient can identify a particular trigger. If the symptoms are mild, a person will try to hold on to or lean against something stable. Often but not always associated with such an attack is anxiety, restlessness, and an urge to bolt from where the attack occurred. Another strong reaction is a fear of impending death. The attack may subside. Its duration can be so brief sometimes that patients can conceal the event from others around them. Such attacks may occur only occasionally or as frequently as a few times a day. Bridges, stairs, empty places, driving a car, or certain social situations typically provoke an attack. Phobic vertigo may follow a period of particular stress or strain. It has been theorized that anxiety itself can cause a certain mismatch of stimuli that results in dizziness.

Depression

Vertigo, light-headedness, and other types of dizziness often occur in depression.

Very often, the depression associated with dizziness is termed "masked depression," because the depressive symptoms may not be present and a person functions well at home, work, or at school. Nevertheless, individuals have a physical symptom—dizziness—that masks the underlying depression.

The causes of clinical depression are not fully understood, but it is known that some people have a hereditary, biological, psychological, or sociological predisposition to it.

Somatization

Some people suffer from a number of vague, multiple physical symptoms for which no cause is found, despite an extensive medical evaluation. Dizziness often plays an important role in these symptoms. Such people are referred to as somatizers, a word that is beginning to replace old terms such as hypochondriac or hysteric. Somatizers are unconsciously expressing a psychological conflict or need. By experiencing the symptoms or becoming preoccupied with finding the cause of them, they are able to repress, alleviate, or divert feelings about whatever is troubling them.

Some somatizers dramatize and even exaggerate their symptoms. For instance, during a neurological examination of gait, the patient may seem to almost topple over, yet that person was able to get to the doctor's office alone by public transportation. Others seem almost unconcerned, even indifferent, to symptoms, but they state that they are very dizzy and are unable to perform many normal activities at home and at work.

Unfortunately, once a person gets a reputation for being a somatizer, family members and primary care physicians don't take their symptoms seriously. If they should develop an illness that is medically treatable, it may not be promptly diagnosed. Somatizers often suffer from a form of depression.

Psychotherapy and Other Treatments

There is no longer any reason to suffer in silence from anxiety and depression. Diagnosis and treatment are available through many sources: community mental health centers, hospital departments of psychiatry, employee assistance programs, outpatient psychiatric clinics and facilities, family social service agencies, and private therapists.

Medication is available to treat depression and anxiety disorders. Only physicians can prescribe medication, but psychotherapy is available from a number of different mental health professionals. Medication and therapy together have been shown to be effective in alleviating many of the symptoms that we have discussed in this chapter. (See also chapter 9.)

PART III

TREATMENT FOR DIZZINESS

Medical, Dietetic, and Surgical Treatments

Millions of people in the United States have experienced dizziness or balance problems. If you or someone you care about is one of these people, it is reassuring to learn there is considerable hope for improvement.

Dizziness is one of the more common reasons for seeking medical care in the over-75 age group. Many older people who have a thorough evaluation learn that deterioration of brain function is the cause of their dizziness. Cure isn't available in the form of a simple pill or surgical procedure, but there are treatments available.

When the cause of dizziness is an underlying systemic disease or allergy, rather than a primary problem of the vestibular system, treatment of the underlying disease will usually reduce or even clear up the dizziness. If you smoke, stop! Smoking can damage arteries and increase the risk of heart disease, stroke, and cancers of the lung, cervix, pancreas, bladder, mouth, and larynx. In addition,

153

smoking can cause, promote, or exacerbate problems with dizziness. Programs available through the American Cancer Society and other groups can help you stop smoking.

When dizziness results from a problem within the vestibular system, or sometimes even in the brain, there are many ways that it can be treated. The treatments fall into several categories, including medication, diet, surgery, physical therapy, and a variety of psychological methods: psychotherapy, visualization, imagery, behavioral methods, biofeedback, and hypnosis.

Medication

A number of drugs work to relieve dizziness, but none of them are perfect. They are successful for some people but often cause uncomfortable, unacceptable side effects. Many other medications can be taken for only short periods of time. Since they can increase the effects of other prescription and nonprescription medications, be sure to tell a doctor about any you already take. Finding the right medication—one that is effective and does not cause undesirable side effects—often depends on dose or frequency, so doctors usually proceed on a trial-and-error basis.

Become involved in your own care. Consult your doctor, pharmacist, or a guidebook to prescription and nonprescription drugs to determine any possible side effects.

Vestibular Suppressants

These drugs have sedative properties, suppress the vestibular system, keeping it from acting up and causing dizziness, but they also cause drowsiness.

Some research studies indicate that vestibular suppressants work by decreasing the firing rate of nerve cells; other reports indicate that this rate increases after patients take the drug for five to seven days.

Vestibular suppressants are indicated for those who suffer severe and lengthy spells of dizziness (an hour or more) or brief spells occurring several times a day.

These drugs reduce the episodes' severity, making them more tolerable, but they do not act as a preventive except in the case of motion sickness. Since severe dizziness often causes vomiting, if you wait to take a pill after the dizziness begins, it may not be retained in the stomach long enough for proper absorption. For this reason, many of the vestibular suppressants come in suppository form and can be taken even after dizziness has begun.

Vestibular suppressants are best for short-term use because of the potential for increased tolerance in some patients. This means that the drugs will not remain effective without increasing the dose, which is undesirable because their sedative properties can impair the brain's ability to learn. Since the brain must learn in order to compensate and overcome the dizziness, the drugs are counterproductive in the long run. True recovery will take longer when you take them, although in the short term the dizziness may be greatly reduced.

One of the most commonly used vestibular suppressants is meclizine (*Antivert, Bonine, Vetrol,* and others). Diphenhydramine (*Benadryl*) and dimenhydrinate (*Dramamine*) are antihistamines used for allergies and sometimes for dizziness. In those people whose allergies may be a primary cause of dizziness, these antihistamines can be effective.

Other drugs that are frequently recommended are the antinausea drugs prochlorperazine (*Compazine*) and promethazine (*Phenergan* and others).

Aside from the common side effect of drowsiness, these drugs produce dry mouth, blurred vision, fast heartbeat, headache, and (paradoxically) insomnia in some people.

Terfenadine (*Seldane*), an antihistamine available by prescription only, has been shown to reduce firing rates of vestibular neurons, but it has not been used much for dizziness. It does have the advantage of not causing drowsiness.

Scopolamine

Scopolamine has become very popular, especially with those who are prone to motion sickness but who still want to enjoy a cruise. This drug and some others fit into a category of their own. They increase heart rate, so they can be considered stimulants, but they induce drowsiness, so they also are considered suppressants. Their beneficial effects on the vestibular function do not seem to relate directly to their sedative properties.

Scopolamine is most often prescribed as a patch, which allows the medication to be absorbed slowly through the skin. The patch is usually placed behind the ear, although it could be placed on any hairless place on the body. (If the skin is thick, as it is in some areas, absorption may be hindered.) Somehow, having it close to the organ of balance seems so logical that most people accept the idea of placing it behind the ear.

Because there are side effects, which can include dry mouth, drowsiness, and sometimes blurred vision, you might want to try using it before you go on a vacation to be sure you are not one of those who experience discomfort with the patch.

Stimulants

Stimulants such as amphetamines and caffeine can alleviate dizziness in some people, but they can make it worse in certain others. In addition, stimulants are known to cause agitation and anxiety. Amphetamines are not prescribed for chronic dizziness because of their addictive qualities, but there is evidence that combining an amphetamine with scopolamine can be very effective for short-term control of motion sickness. The theory behind this is that the side effect of sleepiness caused by the scopolamine is countered by the agitation caused by the amphetamine. It is paradoxical that both stimulants and depressants can accomplish the same thing, reflecting the still-not-understood biochemistry of dizziness.

Antidepressants and Antianxiety Drugs

Dizziness caused by panic attacks or anxiety responds very well to drugs used for those symptoms.

Antidepressants influence nerve cells by altering chemical signals, affecting the rate of metabolism and concentrations of chemicals that pass between the nerves and into the brain. It is not yet clear how these interactions give rise to dizziness or how antidepressants help dizziness in some people. Those people who suffer from both dizziness and depression will feel better, but there is growing evidence that even some people who are not depressed are often helped by these medications.

The simplest class of antidepressants are the tricyclics, thought to affect the transfer of messages between nerve cells. Side effects may include dry mouth, drowsiness, or sexual dysfunction. Among these drugs are amitriptyline (*Elavil* and others), imipramine (*Tofranil*), nortriptyline (*Pamelor*), as well as many others.

Monoamine oxidase (MAO) inhibitors appear to inhibit nerve transmissions in the brain that cause depression. While MAOs are effective in the treatment of depression, it is unclear whether they are also effective in the treatment of dizziness. People who take these drugs need to avoid certain foods; they may also be bothered by the same side effects that are commonly associated with tricyclics.

Other newer drugs that treat depression have not yet been demonstrated to be effective for dizziness. However, when the dizziness is a result of anxiety and/or depression, drugs that control these feelings will also alleviate associated symptoms such as dizziness.

Several drugs, such as alprazolam (*Xanax*) and diazepam (*Valium*), come under the heading of the benzodiazepines. They affect the limbic system, the part of the brain that controls emotions, thus working well against anxiety. These drugs can be effective for dizziness regardless of cause.

Diuretics

These drugs, often referred to as "water pills," are generally used for high blood pressure. They cause excretion in the urine of sodium and potassium, which are referred to as electrolytes. They also relax muscle cells of small arteries. Those with Ménière's disease and other ear disorders often suffer from fluid and salt retention in the inner ear. Thus, dizziness often responds favorably to diuretics.

Side effects are minimal with most diuretics, but it may be recommended that potassium be added, either as part of the diet (orange juice, bananas, etc.) or in pill form. Potassium is essential for normal functioning of the heart, muscles, nerves, and other body organs.

Aminoglycosides

These antibiotics include, among others, streptomycin and gentamicin. Streptomycin was used a great deal in the 1950s to treat tuberculosis and other bacterial ailments. The use of this family of antibiotics today is reserved for certain serious life-threatening infections. These drugs cannot be absorbed if taken orally, so they must be given by injection into the muscles (intramuscularly) or veins (intravenously). They can also be incorporated into ear medications, eyedrops, or ointments used on the skin.

Almost since the introduction of aminoglycosides, it was recognized that large doses could adversely affect the ears, particularly vestibular function. As a result, one theory stated that by giving just enough of these drugs, vestibular function could be destroyed without damaging hearing. The medication is often injected into a muscle at the doctor's office, two or three times a week for two to three weeks. The exact dosage varies from patient to patient. A newer, still experimental treatment consists of administering aminoglycosides by injection or through a tube directly into the ear.

Regardless of how the aminoglycosides are introduced into the body of the person suffering from dizziness, it is always wise and prudent to use the least amount needed. The procedure can be repeated until the desired effect is completed. If the vestibular function (and dizziness) returns later, the treatment can also be repeated. This is much wiser than risking too much of the drug, which can cause hearing loss.

Sometimes this treatment is done in the hospital, where hearing and vestibular function can be closely observed. Regular caloric tests are performed to evaluate vestibular function. Audiometry is also performed to monitor hearing and minimize any risk of hearing loss. Some patients who recover from their severe vertigo are left with a chronic unsteadiness and a temporary illusory feeling that stationary objects are moving back and forth or up and down (oscillopisa).

Aminoglycosides are most often used in people with Ménière's or related problems when both ears experience vestibular effects yet hearing is adequate or good. This is preferable to surgery that may destroy the labyrinth and, with it, hearing.

Other Drugs

Drugs that are used to treat high blood pressure and the cardiovascular system often cause dizziness, but in some cases and in small amounts they may actually treat dizziness.

A drug once commonly used in the treatment of dizziness and other ear disorders is niacin, a B vitamin formerly thought to help dizziness by allowing blood vessels to dilate. Evidence no longer points to its efficacy in influencing blood flow within the ear, so most otolaryngologists no longer recommend it.

When people are thought to have blockages in the blood vessels, medications are often prescribed that can reduce blood coagulation. Aspirin, dipyridamole (*Persantine*), and warfarin (*Coumadin*) are examples of such drugs. However, these drugs will not affect dizziness itself.

If dizziness is associated with migraine headaches, any medication that treats the migraines may be helpful. When migraine headaches and dizziness are associated with the menstrual cycle, medications that reduce body fluid or inflammation may help. These will include diuretics and nonsteroidal anti-inflammatory medications.

When the dizziness is related to a problem within the immune system or results from an autoimmune disease (such as lupus), treatment with steroids and antihistamines is sometimes helpful.

In those cases where there is known vitamin deficiency, vitamin supplements will be useful. Some people in whom there is no such deficiency report that symptoms decrease when they greatly increase their intake of vitamins. However, convincing evidence to support the use of vitamin supplements to treat dizziness is lacking.

TABLE 8.1

USE AND SIDE EFFECTS OF DRUGS FOR TREATMENT
OF DIZZINESS *

• Use: 1=Useless; 10=Very useful
• Side Effects: 1=Many or severe side effects; 10=No side effects.

Sedatives	Use	Side Effects
Meclizine (*Antivert*)	6	7
Prochlorperazine (*Compazine*)	5	5
Promethazine (*Phenergan*)	6	5
Alprazolam (*Xanax*)	7	4
Scopolamine (*Transderm Scōp*)	5	6
Antidepressants		
Amitriptyline (*Elavil*)	3	2
Nortriptyline (*Pamelor*)	3	3

Antidepressants	Use	Side Effects
Tranylcypromine (*Parnate*)	Possibly useful for dizziness and depression in some patients	2
Phenelzine (*Nardil*)	Possibly useful for dizziness and depression in some patients	2

Steroids		
Prednisone (*Deltasone*)	2	Varies with dose and duration
Methylprednisolone (*Medrol*)	2	Varies with dose and duration
Dexamethasone (*Decadron*)	2	Varies with dose and duration

Diuretics		
Hydrochlorothiazide/triamterene (*Dyazide*)	7 for Ménière's disease	7
Hydrochlorothiazide (*HydroDIURIL*)	7 for Ménière's disease	5

Migraine Preparations		
Ergotamine (*Ergostat*)	?	Not yet proven effective for dizziness
Methysergide (*Sansert*)	?	Not yet proven effective for dizziness

Others		
Niacin (*Nicobid*)	2	6
Acetylsalicylic acid (aspirin)	2	2
Betahistine (*Serc*)	1	9
Baclofen (*Lioresal*)	?	Efficacy not established

Others	Use	Side Effects
Warfarin (*Coumadin*)	1	2
		Only used for blood-clotting problems
Dipyridamole (*Persantine*)	1	5
		Only used for blood-clotting problems
Acetazolamide (*Diamox*)	3	4
		for Ménière's disease
Antibiotics	8	3

*Note: These are very general recommendations; not all drugs are appropriate for all individuals and/or all diseases.

Diet

There is some evidence that dizziness can be reduced by altering the inner ear fluid. Substances in the blood and other bodily fluids affect the inner ear fluid. For this reason, changing one's eating habits can be a strong influence.

Lower Dietary Salt

A low-salt diet, especially when combined with diuretics, has been demonstrated to help many people who suffer from Ménière's disease. If you suffer from dizziness from any cause, it is wise not to add salt in cooking or at the table. Avoid (or eat only occasionally and in moderation) salty snacks and foods such as potato chips, salted popcorn, pretzels, crackers, and french fries. Sausage and bacon are especially high in salt, and should also be avoided.

It is not difficult to plan a low-salt diet; your library and local bookstore have books that feature recipes and menus that are either low-salt or salt-free. Look at the sodium content on the package labels. Labels should read "No salt added," "Low in sodium," or "Reduced sodium." Use herbs, spices, and fruit juices to season food. Rinse canned foods such as tuna and vegetables to remove salty juices.

Avoid Caffeine

Caffeine is another substance that can exacerbate or promote dizziness. Because caffeine constricts the blood vessels, circulation to the inner ear may also be reduced. Many people report that their dizziness increases when they are anxious or agitated. Since caffeine is a stimulant, it is not surprising that those who ingest a great deal of it experience dizziness. The dizziness experienced as a result of excessive caffeine intake itself is usually a feeling of lightheadedness or vague imbalance, and is rarely disabling. It is not to be confused with turning or vertigo.

Caffeine is, of course, found in coffee, but tea and cocoa also have a high content of caffeine or similar substances. Brewed coffee usually has more caffeine in it than instant coffee does. Many carbonated beverages, especially cola drinks, also contain caffeine. Chocolate contains a substance similar to caffeine and with much the same effects. Some over-the-counter medications contain caffeine, so it is wise to avoid them.

It may be difficult to eliminate caffeine from your diet, especially if you are in the habit of drinking several cups of coffee or cola drinks each day. If possible, try to cut down gradually. You might want to alternate decaffeinated coffee and cola with your usual caffeinated drink. If you suddenly eliminate caffeine, you may experience withdrawal symptoms such as headaches and tiredness. Try to endure this for a few days; you may find that your dizziness is improved.

Cut Back on Sugar

Although research on sugar's role in causing dizziness is not impressive, there are doctors who believe that high sugar levels in the blood may increase vestibular problems. There are two forms of sugar: simple and complex (carbohydrates such as starches, grains, pasta, peas and other vegetables). The latter are digested gradually, and nutrients released into the bloodstream are not very likely to affect the inner ear.

Simple sugars, on the other hand, consist of table sugar, brown sugar, honey, molasses, and corn syrup, all of which are quickly broken down and released into the bloodstream. The body may use this sugar immediately for energy, so much of the body's blood sugar is quickly depleted. Some researchers have suggested that this fluctuation in blood sugar levels may cause some changes in inner ear fluids, promoting dizziness in those people who already have a problem.

If you are willing to test this hypothesis, choose a sugar substitute for your diet. Many prepared foods and beverages are made with sugar substitutes. Substituting fruit for cake and other sweets, mixing club soda with fruit juice to make your own carbonated drinks, and trying some naturally sweet herbal teas all can help satisfy your sweet tooth without raising your blood sugar.

Other Tips

Avoid foods containing monosodium glutamate (MSG) because they contain sodium, which may increase your symptoms. Limit alcohol intake, even though in moderation it may serve as a relaxant and dilate the arteries. Alcohol can cause unsteadiness in any amounts.

Eating, snacking, and drinking fluids at regular times helps to maintain bodily fluids at a constant level, which also keeps the inner ear fluid stable.

It is possible that a particular food may cause allergies for some people. Foods that are most likely to cause such symptoms are milk, tomatoes, oranges, fish, and mushrooms. Allergies are sometimes related to dizziness, especially in those people for whom there is no specific finding. For this reason, it is wise to avoid any foods that you think might be responsible for such episodes. Keep a food diary, noting what and when you eat, and also make a note of when you experience dizziness. If a pattern emerges associating particular foods or a class of foods with episodes of dizziness, try avoiding those foods for a while. If your dizziness improves, you may have discovered an important relationship. You can, at some later time, try to reintroduce the offending food in small quantities to determine if the relationship persists.

Are there any foods that might particularly alleviate dizziness? None have been proven to do so, although many people have favorites that calm them down during dizzy episodes. Herbal teas might be good for some people, crackers and juice for others. Still others find just sipping water helpful.

Surgery

An entire range of surgical procedures has been developed for certain vestibular conditions, especially Ménière's disease. For the most part, surgery has been overutilized as a treatment for dizziness. Most people recover from damage to their vestibular systems whether or not they have surgery.

The surgical procedures described on the following pages are done in a hospital operating room. Some procedures are performed under general anesthesia, in which the patient is fully asleep; others are carried out under local anesthesia, in which the patient usually has some sort of numbing injection in the area of the surgery. In addition, sedation is usually offered by injection into a muscle or vein. Depending on the procedure and the state of the patient's health, time spent in the hospital will vary.

Recuperation after surgery depends on many factors, but don't expect improvement in symptoms for six to eight weeks or even longer.

Choosing a Surgeon

If you are considering having surgery for dizziness, it is important that your surgeon be board certified in the specialty of otolaryngology and, in some instances, neurosurgery. To become board certified, a physician must complete an accredited residency in a hospital and pass a rigorous examination given by one of the 24 specialty boards recognized by the American Board of Medical Specialties (ABMS). Your library is a good place to find a list of such physicians in your own area. Ask the librarian about consulting the Directory of Medical Specialists. To find out if a particular doctor is certified, you can also consult the directory or call the ABMS hot line at 800-776-2378. You might also want to ask the doctor if he or she is experienced performing the procedure, but keep in mind that any doctor who says "I do them all the time" may be doing many unnecessary procedures.

Deciding on the Hospital

Usually, board-certified physicians are associated with good hospitals, but there are still some things you can do to reassure yourself that you will be in a hospital with a good track record.

A hospital should be accredited by the Joint Commission on Accreditation of Healthcare Organizations (JCOAH). This indicates that the hospital has met rigorous standards, so avoid any that are not JCOAH accredited.

Types of Surgery

There are two categories of surgery that are done on people who suffer from dizziness: destructive and nondestructive procedures. The destructive procedures deliberately destroy or allow destruction of hearing and/or vestibular function. This is usually done when both vestibular and hearing function are already severely impaired. The nondestructive procedures are meant to conserve hearing, but Ménière's and other diseases may progress so that hearing may continue to deteriorate over time in spite of surgery for vertigo.

Nondestructive Procedures

ENDOLYMPHATIC SAC SURGERY. This is probably the most common type of surgery performed for Ménière's disease. The endolymphatic duct empties into an area surrounding the brain. In Ménière's disease, it is thought that the endolymphatic fluid is either overproduced or not absorbed well enough back into the body, causing swelling of the endolymphatic compartment of the inner ear. The idea behind this operation is to drain this fluid.

There are several variations of the surgical procedure. One method is to place a drain from the endolymphatic sac into the mastoid cavity. The mastoid cavity is the bone behind the ear and is normally filled with small openings like a bee's honeycomb. It can become infected, and in the days before antibiotics, this often happened to children. In Ménière's disease, the mastoid is usually normal. Nevertheless, in this procedure, the air cells or openings are removed, exposing bone overlying the brain behind the inner ear. This bone is gently removed so that the tissue covering the brain and the endolymphatic sac come into view. An incision can then be made in the sac, and one of several plastic devices is placed so that it drains fluid into the mastoid or into the cerebrospinal fluid on the other side of the sac. Some surgeons placed a sheet of plastic in the sac, which remains there, draining the fluid into either the mastoid or the cerebrospinal fluid.

It seems logical that surgically draining this fluid would help relieve the patient's dizziness, but for various reasons—some understood and others not—the results of the surgery are often disappointing. For this reason, many ear surgeons have abandoned the procedure. Nevertheless, some surgeons are still enthusiastic about it. Many patients report that the operation was a tremendous success, one that made a significant difference in the quality of their lives.

The risks of this operation, as with any ear operation, include the possibility of damage to the facial nerve, exacerbation of the dizziness, hearing loss, and infection. These complications seldom occur when the surgery is performed by an experienced surgeon. The procedure itself is usually done under general anesthesia, and it lasts about three hours. Expect to be hospitalized overnight.

TACK OPERATION. In this nondestructive operation, an actual metal tack is placed through the foot plate of the stapes bone so that the tip of the tack protrudes into the inner ear. The idea is that when the saccule distends, as it does in Ménière's disease, it will burst and rupture like a balloon when it encounters the sharp end of the tack. Thus, severe vertigo does not develop. However, this procedure is not recommended because there is some doubt about its efficacy. Moreover, loss of hearing is likely to occur. The procedure itself takes about one hour under general anesthesia and necessitates an overnight stay in a hospital.

COCHLEOSACCULOTOMY. This operation is performed for Ménière's disease. A small instrument with a sharp edge is used to pierce the inner ear through the round window in such a manner that the utricle is penetrated. The hope is to relieve pressure in the inner ear and thereby relieve Ménière's disease. It is possible that the fluid will accumulate again, but the proponents of the procedure say this is not a problem.

Although this is considered a nondestructive procedure, many patients will experience hearing loss after it. It is useful for elderly patients because it is quicker than others and may give enough relief to make a patient more comfortable. The procedure itself takes about one hour, and can be done under local or general anesthesia. Hospitalization is usually overnight.

PERILYMPH FISTULA SURGERY. Perilymph fistula is difficult to diagnose, even at surgery when a leak of fluid is seen in the middle ear. During this procedure a piece of fat or tissue surrounding muscle is placed into the oval and/or round windows. This is supposed to stop the leak, but of course it may also impair the vibration of the ossicles and reduce hearing. Many of these pieces of tissue fall out. There is serious doubt as to whether this operation is useful. The surgeon-author of this book would not have it done on himself for dizziness and would not recommend it. The procedure takes about an hour, and is done as an outpatient. Recovery time is seven to ten days.

Younger and/or healthier patients usually have better results from the destructive procedures described below.

Although physicians who are enthusiastic about nondestructive procedures claim great success for curing vertigo, it is the opinion of many otolaryngologists that the diagnosis may have been incorrect and that the vertigo would have disappeared on its own, without any of these "cures."

Destructive Procedures

LABYRINTHECTOMY. This procedure is one of the oldest that is performed for Ménière's disease and other vestibular disorders involving the ear. There are several forms of the operation, but essentially they all destroy the labyrinth and, therefore, all hearing and balance function in that ear.

The most common procedure is one in which the ear is opened and the semicircular canals are drilled away. This destroys both the vestibular and hearing part of the inner ear. If hearing loss is already severe, as it often is with Ménière's disease, labyrinthectomy may be a good choice, but if hearing in the involved ear is quite good, it is not usually recommended.

A variation of the labyrinthectomy is to drill the bone between the oval and round windows, thereby connecting them. This destroys the inner ear. It is quicker and less disabling than many other procedures, so many surgeons recommend it for their elderly patients. There is always total loss of hearing with this procedure. It appears not to be as successful as other procedures at stopping the dizziness over long periods of time, though, because the neural structures of the inner ear can partially recover. A complete labyrinthectomy usually attains better results, and in the surgeon-author's opinion, is preferable.

Many surgeons also place a little bit of streptomycin in the ear. This antibiotic is destructive to vestibular function. It is often effective, but there is also evidence that vestibular function can be restored to a small extent. It may take over a year to occur, but the result might be dizziness. The hope is that the streptomycin will kill any remaining hair cells, thus avoiding or forestalling regeneration of the vestibular system.

Both of these procedures take about three hours under general anesthesia. The patient is usually hospitalized overnight.

A streptomycin perfusion operation is also advocated by some ear surgeons. This involves irrigation of the inner ear with streptomycin during an operation. Advocates claim that this perfusion does not harm hearing at all, but destroys vestibular function, as one might suspect; however, others that try the operation find that flushing the delicate labyrinth of the inner ear does affect hearing adversely. There does not appear to be a significant advantage in giving streptomycin directly into the ear during a large operation over injecting it through a tube or needle through the eardrum as an outpatient. The optimal dose of the drug is not known for any individual so that the operation is a one-shot guess. In the outpatient setting the procedure can be repeated as many times as needed in order to obtain the response desired. The operation takes two to three hours, requires overnight hospital stay, and has a recuperation time of two weeks.

VESTIBULAR NERVE SECTION. When dizziness is incapacitating and disabling but hearing is intact, cutting the vestibular nerve between the brain and the ear can bring significant relief from spells of vertigo. This procedure results in the ear having no vestibular function.

The incision is made either from above or behind the ear. Technically challenging, the procedure is successful in the hands of an experienced surgeon.

This is major surgery, however, taking about four hours under general anesthesia. The brain must be eased out of the way to perform the procedure, so both an otolaryngologist, and a neurosurgeon will be involved in the surgery. The patient generally must spend time in the intensive care unit following the operation, and must stay in the hospital a total of five to seven days.

Risks include infection, meningitis, hearing loss, facial nerve paralysis, stroke, and seizures. On a more optimistic note, if done by experienced and qualified surgeons, the chance of any of these side effects is low.

Following the surgery, there is often a period of severe dizziness. This occurs because the vestibular information from the opposite side of the body has been totally removed and the brain must now adjust. The normal brain learns to compensate, and the dizziness ceases. For most people, if there was poor vestibular function in the operated ear before surgery, there should be less dizziness. The reason for this is that often patients have just enough function in the ear to cause dizziness, and once the function is totally destroyed, their spells of dizziness cease.

Elderly patients or those in whom the brain plays a contributory role in dizziness often cannot compensate fully. Therefore, prior to performing the operation, it is extremely important to confirm that the ear, and not the brain, is the actual cause of the dizziness.

Cutting the vestibular nerve on both sides would cause a serious balance and walking disability, because there would essentially be no vestibular function. For this reason, the procedure is done on only one side. Obviously, if both ears are involved in causing the dizziness, this would not be an appropriate operation. In people with Ménière's disease, only one ear is usually involved, but sometimes the other ear does become affected later. If this occurs, the dizziness would naturally recur, and the patient would be even worse off than prior to the surgery.

As a result of these effects, the operation is usually reserved for those whose disability from vertigo is severe and of long duration. It is unlikely to improve constant imbalance or other forms of dizziness.

Despite some of the negative factors relating to this surgery, it is the single most effective operation for control of severe spells of vertigo.

OTHER DESTRUCTIVE PROCEDURES. There are other operations that combine some of the procedures already discussed. The vestibular nerve can be cut, for example, by going through the cochlea or through the vestibular portion of the ear. The incision is made behind the ear. Some surgeons combine the labyrinthectomy and vestibular nerve section because they feel that this approach is most effective in destroying the function of the inner ear. It is always possible that a few nerve fibers could be left over after cutting the vestibular nerve, or that some fibers could regrow and provide some abnormal vestibular function after labyrinthectomy. The combined approach possibly reduces the chance of recurrence of either of these two complications. These combined procedures might be called transcochlear vestibular nerve section or translabyrinthine vestibular nerve section. They take about three hours under general anesthesia. Hospitalization is usually overnight.

Specialized Procedures

VASCULAR LOOP SURGERY. Another new type of surgery for Ménière's disease or other diseases is usually performed by neurosurgeons. It is based on the theory that loops of blood vessels inside the head are pushing on the vestibular nerve and causing irritation. Surgeons who advocate this surgery believe that by placing a piece of felt or other material between the nerve and the offending blood vessel, the patient will be relieved of symptoms. This theory is based on other procedures in which it is known that blood vessels are pushing on nerves.

In this instance, however, it is not possible to tell if there is a blood vessel pressing on the nerve. Even the most accurate CT scans or magnetic resonance imaging (MRI) cannot differentiate these small structures inside the head. Since blood vessels are always in the area of the vestibular nerve, it is impossible, in this surgeon's opinion, to know if one of these vessels is doing any damage. Nevertheless, some surgeons say that there are various tests that can determine the difference between dysfunction of the nerve and a vessel pressing on the nerve and causing damage.

Not only is there doubt about the rationale for this operation, but the procedure takes about four to five hours under general anesthesia. The patient must remain in the hospital five to ten days, and recuperation at home takes 21 to 30 days. More important, this procedure carries much more risk of meningitis, stroke, or even death than standard approaches. It is not recommended by the surgeon-author of this book.

SURGERY FOR BPPV. Surgery is sometimes performed for people whose benign paroxysmal positional vertigo is severe and disabling and has persisted with no remission for over a year. This procedure involves cutting a nerve in the semicircular canal of the ear. The operation is usually done by making an incision in the ear canal lifting up the skin of the ear canal, and going under the eardrum. The singular nerve that transmits nerve impulses from the posterior semicircular canal is found near the round window. Bone is drilled away, and the nerve is located and cut.

This is a very challenging operation, although it takes only one hour under general anesthesia and requires overnight hospitalization. The main risk of this procedure is hearing loss. Facial nerve injury, infection, and other problems related to ear surgery may occur, but these are less likely.

An interesting new procedure that has been developed for BPPV is to divide the posterior semicircular canal. The hope is that this will prevent the endolymph from flowing, one of the causes of the dizziness. It is too soon to tell how effective this procedure is.

MYRINGOTOMY AND TYMPANOSTOMY TUBES. This is a surgical approach used for ear infections that, incidentally, also helps dizziness. An incision is made into the eardrum (myringotomy), sometimes to drain an acutely infected ear. Then, tiny hollow tubes are usually inserted into the eardrum, allowing continuous draining of fluid. The tubes remain in, but come out spontaneously 6 to 18 months later. This can reduce the imbalance and mild turning that some patients experience along with the infection. The procedure removes the fluid, keeping it from reaccumulating and reducing the hearing loss that accompanies the condition.

The procedure takes only about 15 minutes and can be done under local anesthesia in adults (but requires general anesthesia in children). Overnight hospitalization usually isn't needed.

STAPEDECTOMY. This operation is sometimes done for perilymph fistula. It is not recommended by most otolaryngologists, including the surgeon-author of this book.

Stapedectomy is very useful, however, to help restore hearing when *otosclerosis* has developed in one ear. Otosclerosis is a condition in which the bones of hearing, ossicles in the middle ear, become fixed. This impedes the stapes from vibrating properly, thus causing hearing loss and noise in the ear (tinnitus).

There are several procedures that can be done, most of which involve removing all or part of the stapes bone and covering the opening into the inner ear with a tiny graft, usually body fat tissue taken directly from behind the patient's ear. The end of a piece of wire is wrapped around the graft and the other end is attached to one hearing bone (the incus) of the middle ear. This surgery tends to be very successful in patients whose hearing loss is due to otosclerosis. As with any ear surgery, complications can occur, and the perilymph can leak around the graft.

The procedure itself takes one hour, and most often is done on an outpatient basis in an operating room at the hospital. Some patients may stay overnight. The operation is usually done under local anesthesia.

Most of the surgical procedures that have been discussed here are directed against Ménière's disease. There is good reason for this. Other vestibular diseases such as vestibular neuronitis, infections, or other problems may result in significant damage to the vestibular nerve, making such surgery unnecessary. The disease becomes chronic, and the patient compensates and recovers. (Certain exercises and other therapeutic approaches useful for dizziness will be discussed in chapter 9.)

There is no surgical approach that is reasonable for dizziness alone when it is associated with a vestibular disorder involving the brain. Surgery is often indicated for certain tumors or problems, such as an accumulation of fluid in the brain, that may have associated dizziness. But dizziness alone is never a reason to undergo brain surgery.

However, if the disease that is causing dizziness is confined to the inner ear itself and creating a major disability for the patient, surgery certainly should be considered.

The Value of Dizziness Surgery

ONE SURGEON'S OPINION BASED ON THE QUESTION,
"IF I WERE THE PATIENT, WOULD I HAVE THIS OPERATION?"
ASSUMING THAT THE PROPER DISEASE IS PRESENT

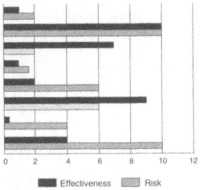

9

Therapy and Rehabilitation

There are many other approaches to treating dizziness besides medication, diet, and surgery, and you may already be using them. For instance, many people spontaneously develop habits that attempt to block out the sensory input that is causing them trouble: If they are prone to acute, severe imbalance episodes because of a problem with the inner ear, they hold their heads as still as possible while performing their daily activities. At the dinner table, they refrain from turning toward the person who is speaking, relying instead on just listening. They worry that their vestibular systems won't help them regain their balance if they stumble, so they become very vision-oriented, increasing the sensory input that comes from sight and watching carefully to make sure they haven't missed a step. If their muscles and joints are giving them trouble, they recognize that they can't depend on getting information from those sensors either, so they rely more heavily on vision and perhaps the use of a cane.

Sometimes these are wise moves, but wouldn't it be better to fix the source of the sensory input that isn't up to par?

You have probably found that when something is difficult or makes you uncomfortable, you try to do it anyway, starting perhaps in small steps. Eventually, you become used to it. This sort of "desensitization" can work for dizziness. In addition to, or instead of, medication and surgery, certain planned activities and physical therapy can reduce or even eliminate dizziness. These techniques are especially useful for dizziness caused by positional changes, because the brain can learn to adapt to certain positions.

More and more, the medical profession is taking a team approach to dizziness. Although your first line of help comes from your doctor, other professionals may also become involved.

Team Approach to Rehabilitation

In addition to physicians who treat dizziness or underlying medical conditions, other professionals who may have a role in your rehabilitation include physical therapists, occupational therapists, nurses, eye care professionals, speech and hearing therapists, nutritionists and dietitians, pharmacists, and mental health professionals, including psychiatrists, psychologists, and social workers. Together, their goals are to reduce the frequency and duration of your dizziness and to improve your balance while walking.

Physical Therapists

Physical therapists hold at least an undergraduate degree in physical therapy and are licensed in the state in which they practice. They assist in the examination, testing, and treatment of people who are temporarily or permanently physically disabled. They work in hospitals and nursing homes, and also join home-care teams. Some physical therapists have their own offices, treating people who have been referred to them by physicians. Goals vary according to the physical potential and age of the patient, but a return to functioning as normally as possible is always the ultimate objective of physical therapy.

Based on information available from other professionals who have evaluated the patient, physical therapists who are familiar with vestibular issues can offer a wide range of exercises and activities. If problems with dizziness are related to vestibular deficits, exercises (such as the ones described later) are demonstrated, and you will be guided toward mastery. A physical therapist, working in collaboration with your physician or others, may give you an individualized plan to help your brain learn to overcome the dizziness that was caused by certain positions of the head.

Some patients, particularly older ones, have balance and dizziness problems that are only partly caused by lack of vestibular function. They may be suffering from generalized weakness, arthritis (particularly of the neck or the feet and legs), or simply degeneration of a number of the body's functions. Certain strengthening exercises and general conditioning can help such people regain some lost function.

Regardless of your age and general condition, physical therapists can help set up a program that is appropriate for you. It may be as simple as a few very brief walks each day, or as extensive as weight-bearing exercises, bicycle riding, or calisthenics.

If, for instance, you have been overtaxing your eyes to compensate for your vestibular problems, the major focus will be on retraining your balance system. You may practice walking on deep pile carpeting or pillows, and eventually on a balance beam. If your hand-to-eye coordination is limited, a simple game of catch may be difficult at first, but eventually you will increase your skills. You may be encouraged to play video games, which can improve hand-to-eye coordination.

Some physical therapists may also be familiar with relaxation techniques and other ways of helping people overcome dizziness.

Occupational Therapists

Occupational therapists have at least an undergraduate degree and are licensed in the state in which they practice. They may also be part of the team that works with patients trying to overcome dizziness. Occupational therapists use purposeful, specific activity with people whose ability to function independently is limited for any number of reasons, including physical injury or illness. If they are familiar with treatments for dizziness, they can often help patients learn alternative ways to achieve and maintain independence, even if a return to the patients' original level of functioning is not a reachable goal. Occupational therapists work in hospitals and other institutions, and are often part of a home-care team.

In any of these settings, occupational therapists try to help you do as much for yourself as possible. Often, they accomplish this with the aid of various adaptive equipment, such as canes, walkers, and raised chair or toilet seats, or by changing the patient's environment at home, in the workplace, and elsewhere. They may suggest that patients rearrange furniture, or increase the light in and around the home to improve visual cues; they may also recommend ways to make reading more comfortable.

Nurses

Nurses are educated at different levels. Some are graduates of nursing schools, whereas others have advanced degrees. They, too, are licensed in the state in which they practice. Nurses may be involved with patients from the time of evaluation through treatment. Many assist physicians in a number of tasks, and are the professionals who give hands-on care, especially during hospitalization. They have an important role as teachers as well, instructing patients in self-care and making certain that they have understood all of the doctor's instructions.

Eye Care Professionals

Eye care professionals include ophthalmologists (physicians who specialize in evaluation, treatment, and surgery of the eyes), optometrists, and opticians. They may recommend ways to enhance or improve the patient's visual input, perhaps with certain kinds of eyeglasses that allow increased light to reach the eyes. Nonreflective lenses and larger frames can be helpful.

Some dizziness, particularly when related to motion sickness, may be visually induced rather than caused by vestibular stimuli. This is the kind of dizziness that occurs when you watch a movie involving a great deal of motion, or look at a train that is passing by quickly. Trying to keep your eye on the ball while watching a tennis match, regardless of where you are seated, can also cause this kind of dizziness. If your dizziness is due to a mismatch of stimuli, exercises in which your eyes (and thus you) slowly become accustomed to watching a moving object can be helpful.

Speech and Hearing Therapists

Speech and hearing therapists, sometimes called speech and hearing pathologists, have at least an undergraduate degree and are usually registered or licensed in their state. They are trained to treat people with communication disorders. If you have severe or even mild hearing loss as well as dizziness, or if dizziness has limited your ability to read or is the result of a neurological problem, they can help you regain your ability to read and communicate orally.

Nutritionists and Dietitians

Although we discussed diet in the previous chapter, if you are seeking additional advice on good nutrition, you may wish to consult with a specialist. Since anyone can call himself/herself a nutritionist, you should check qualifications. Registered dietitians hold at least an undergraduate degree, have been trained in the principles of sound nutrition, and are certified by the American Dietetic Association. Nutritionists, who also hold at least an undergraduate degree, are usually members of one of the major nutrition associations. Ask your physician or another trusted professional to recommend a competent nutritional expert to you.

Pharmacists

These are professionals who have intensive, ongoing training in the preparation and dispensation of medications. In choosing a pharmacy for your medication needs at home, find one that keeps track of all the drugs (prescription and nonprescription) that you use. Most pharmacies now have computers so that they can efficiently maintain your medication profile. In this way, they can make sure that you are using your drugs correctly and that there is no risk of any harmful interaction between them. This is important, because some drugs given for purposes other than dizziness can exacerbate your symptoms and counteract medication for the dizziness. Pharmacists are also a good source of information about side effects and symptoms that should be reported to your physician as well as about interactions of drugs with food, proper timing of doses, and special storage requirements.

Mental Health Professionals

Psychiatrists are physicians trained in the causes, treatment, and prevention of mental, emotional, and behavioral problems and disorders. Many specialize in the relationship between physical disease and emotions, and can prescribe medication when indicated. A psychiatrist should be board eligible or certified in that specialty.

Psychologists have a master's degree or doctorate in psychology. They are licensed in the state in which they practice. They can offer counseling and short- or long-term psychotherapy, and many make a specialty of working with patients who have medical as well as emotional problems. *Social workers* usually have a master's degree or doctorate in social work. Some have a bachelor's degree or work as social work aides. Generally, they aim to enhance the relationships between individuals and their environment or surroundings. Medical social workers are usually familiar with the physical and psychological aspects of illnesses. Those with graduate degrees are trained to provide short-term or even intensive long-term counseling. If they are in private practice, they should be certified or licensed in the state in which they practice. Social workers at all levels of education are usually involved in helping patients at the time of their discharge from a hospital, and these professionals are often an integral part of a rehabilitation team.

Any of the therapists listed previously will, either individually or together, help you with a program of planned activities that includes physical therapy, dietary changes, psychological counseling, and methods such as relaxation techniques and biofeedback. You will do exercises with the physical therapist, but you will also be given "homework" to do on your own.

If your dizziness is mild, or if for some reason you are unable to consult with a rehabilitation team, there are a number of exercises that you can do on your own. They constitute a major part of the treatment for dizziness.

Physical Therapy Exercises You Can Do at Home

The aim of the following exercises is to help you to:
- train your eye movements to be independent of your head
- practice balance
- practice the very head movements that cause dizziness so that the brain learns to compensate

- loosen up muscles that are causing spasms in your neck and contributing to dizziness
- improve general mobility
- build self-confidence as you find that your dizziness becomes more manageable

Follow the simple instructions below, being careful not to try to do too much at a time. Before you begin, ask someone to be with you so that if you become dizzy, you are not at risk of falling. If progress is slow, don't become discouraged. It can take a considerable amount of time for the brain to learn to overcome dizziness.

Eye and Head Coordination Exercises

These exercises are for improving eye coordination. Do each exercise 15 to 20 times, three times a day.

1. EYE COORDINATION.

Step 1. Sit in a comfortable chair with arms.
Step 2. With head held still and your eyes open, look up, then down, at first slowly, then increasing the speed.
Step 3. With head held still and your eyes open, look from one side to the other, at first slowly, then increasing the speed.
Step 4. With head held still, focus on a finger held at arm's length, slowly moving it as close to your nose as you can focus, then move it away to arm's length.

2. HEAD AND EYE MOVEMENTS.

Do each step with your eyes open, but as you begin to improve, repeat the steps with eyes closed.
Step 1. Sit in a comfortable chair with arms.
Step 2. Bend your head forward, then backward, at first slowly, then increasing the speed.
Step 3. Turn your head from side to side, at first slowly, then increasing the speed.

Postural Control Exercises

These exercises are designed to improve balance while walking. They are listed in approximate order of difficulty.

Begin with the first one, continuing on to the two or three that you find most difficult. When these become easier, go on to the next three.

You should do these exercises three times a day. Do each one for 30 seconds on a bare floor, lightweight carpeting, or stable rug, but avoid thick-pile carpets. Do the exercises barefoot or wear shoes with thin, flat soles.

Each exercise should be done first with your eyes open, then repeated with eyes closed.

1. Stand on the floor with both feet together.
2. Stand with one foot ahead of the other, the heel touching the toe.
3. Walk, using a steady, narrow gait and with your feet closely side by side.
4. Walk slowly, feet straight, so that the heel of one foot touches the toe of the other with each step.
5. Walk slowly, moving your head quickly back and forth as far to the right and left as you can.
6. Stand on one foot at a time. While standing, move the other foot forward and backward, as far as you can, without touching the floor.

Brain Recall Exercise

In this exercise, the goal is to help the brain remember where a target is with the eyes closed. Practice it for about two or three minutes, three times a day.

Step 1. Choose two objects in the room that are far apart, but close enough so that you can see them by moving your eyes but not your head. One object should be high and the other low. You might choose a plant, light switch, doorknob, picture on the wall, or any other suitable object.

Step 2. Move your head and eyes so that you are looking directly at one of the objects. Then close your eyes and move your head so that when you open your eyes, they will be perfectly positioned on the second object.

Step 3. Open your eyes and look at the second object. Pay careful attention to where your eyes looked at the moment you opened them. Note if you have to move your eyes to find the second object.

Repeat this exercise, sometimes looking first at one object and other times the other, until you have trained your brain so well that you find the second object as soon as you open your eyes.

Change the objects and locations as you progress, using objects so far apart that you must move your head as well as your eyes to see them. Continue this exercise until you are able to do this competently.

Exercises for Benign Paroxysmal Positional Vertigo (BPPV)

These exercises are similar to those done to evaluate dizziness. Repeat them three times in each exercise session. Do three to four sessions a day.

1. LYING-DOWN EXERCISES. Lie down with your head hanging over the end of a couch, bed, or other surface.
Step 1. Turn your head so that your right ear points toward the floor. This may make you dizzy. Hold this position for 10 to 20 seconds, or until dizziness subsides.
Step 2. Move your head back to the initial position.
Step 3. Turn your head so that your left ear points toward the floor. This may also make you dizzy. Hold this position for 10 to 20 seconds, or until dizziness subsides.

2. SITTING-DOWN EXERCISES. These are more difficult than the lying-down exercises, and are even more likely to make you dizzy. For this reason, sit on a chair with arms, a couch, or the middle of the bed so you will not fall down if you become dizzy.
Step 1. Sit in an upright position.
Step 2. Bend quickly at the waist, as far to the right side as you can, so that your head is hanging way over to the right. Hold this position for 20 seconds, then sit up.

Step 3. Bend quickly at the waist, as far to the left side as you can, so that your head is hanging way over to the left. Hold this position for 20 seconds, then sit up.

HEAD ROTATION EXERCISES.
These exercises are designed to stimulate the balance sensors in the inner ear. They are likely to cause dizziness because the goal is to train your vestibular system to adapt to movements that cause dizziness. They are also excellent for limbering up shoulder muscles and any other muscles that seem tight. These, too, should be done while sitting in a chair with arms or the middle of a bed (or any other safe place) so that you don't fall if you feel very dizzy.

Repeat the exercises two to three times in each session. Do three sessions each day.

1. HORIZONTAL HEAD ROTATIONS.
Step 1. In a seated position, look forward.
Step 2. Rotate your head all the way to the right and then all the way to the left, going back and forth. Start slowly and increase the speed of rotation of your head as much as you can. Do this for 20 seconds.

2. VERTICAL HEAD ROTATIONS.
Step 1. In a seated position, look forward.
Step 2. Turn your head to the right so that you are 45 degrees (one-eighth of a circle) from the position in Step 1.
Step 3. Move the top of your head so that your left ear moves toward the left knee.
Step 4. Return your head to the position in Step 2.
Step 5. Continue to alternate positions in Step 3 and Step 4 as quickly as you can for 20 seconds.
Step 6. Still in a seated position, look forward.
Step 7. Turn your head to the left so that you are 45 degrees (one-eighth of a circle) from the position in Step 6.
Step 8. Move the top of your head so that your right ear moves in the direction of the right knee.

Step 9. Return your head to the position in Step 7.

Step 10. Continue to alternate positions in Step 8 and Step 9 as quickly as you can for 20 seconds.

Relaxation Techniques

When you are plagued with dizzy spells, you may have many fears. Will you be able to work or return to former relationships and activities? Will you need surgery? Will you ever feel better? All of this can cause negative stress, making you feel as though you lack control over your life and are unable to cope. The rest of this chapter will outline some techniques that are not standard, but may help some people who have undergone a thorough evaluation without significant abnormality detected.

Now is a good time to learn techniques that provide a means of achieving muscle and mind relaxation. This can shift attention away from anxiety, dizziness, and other symptoms that often interact to exacerbate every sensation. Relaxation techniques can reduce symptoms, increase coping skills, and enhance the quality of your life. Many psychologists, social workers, nurses, physical therapists, and other health professionals use relaxation methods as part of their treatment, and those on your rehabilitation team may be able to teach them to you or recommend someone who can.

If you can't find a professional to work with, make use of audiotapes. Begin by listening in a quiet spot, using earphones so that all distractions are blocked out. As you become more accustomed to these techniques, you will want to do them in different settings. Eventually, you will be able to use the techniques without outside guidance (instructor or tape), and will begin to relax even in a noisy, busy setting.

There are two kinds of relaxation techniques—passive relaxation and progressive relaxation—that are most commonly recommended.

Passive Relaxation

Passive relaxation is similar to self-hypnosis or meditation because its purpose is to achieve a state of deep relaxation. Through instruction, you can enter this relaxed state and pay attention to the sensation in different muscle groups, from your feet up to your head. The person guiding you in this technique may suggest you visualize certain tranquil images, such as a quiet, blue sea or a snow-covered mountain. You are encouraged to consider your own appealing scene, perhaps one that is familiar to you. These images or scenes help to sustain a relaxed mood, distracting you from stressful scenes or thoughts. At the end of the session, you will be encouraged to open your eyes slowly and become alert.

You can do the following simple exercise yourself without benefit of outside help.

- Choose a word that evokes a quiet, calm feeling. Examples might be a color, an object, or simply the word "sky," "sea," "peace," or anything that suits you.
- Slowly and deeply inhale, counting up to five. Between each count, say the word you chose quietly to yourself.
- Hold your breath for one second. Slowly exhale, counting again either forward or backward. Silently or very quietly, repeat your chosen word.
- Relax your chest and stomach muscles and drop your shoulders.
- Repeat three to five times.

Progressive Relaxation

Progressive relaxation includes some of the techniques of passive relaxation, including breathing and imagery. This technique differs in that it involves the tensing and relaxing of specific muscle groups. By tensing the muscles before relaxing them, some proponents believe you achieve a greater degree of relaxation. Some typical exercises include making a fist and then relaxing the hand, or curling the toes of a foot and then relaxing the foot. It is usually suggested that you start with hands and feet, moving up the body and ending with the face, eyes, and head. These, too, can be taught to you in person or through an audiotape or book.

Hypnosis

Some people still think of hypnosis as a parlor trick or theatrical experience, yet it has long had a place as an adjunct to psychotherapy. It can accelerate the impact of psychotherapeutic interventions and can also be a primary method of dealing with certain problems.

A hypnotist-therapist creates an atmosphere of security and relaxation, then helps you enter a passive, trancelike state. This resembles normal sleep, during which perception and memory are altered, permitting you to respond to suggestions. Hypnosis is also described as a form of arousal or focused concentration during which there is no awareness of what is going on around you, where you are, or what time it is. Suggestions for the posthypnotic period can also be made during hypnosis.

Because hypnosis allows the mind to ignore involuntary body responses, awareness of pain or discomfort can be blocked and replaced with more positive feelings. Many psychotherapists encourage people to consider hypnosis if they are experiencing uncomfortable side effects, such as the nausea associated with chemotherapy. Hypnosis is also useful in controlling habits such as smoking or nail biting. The therapist uses the patient's intense focus to guide him or her to change behaviors, attitudes, or ways of coping.

Self-hypnosis, sometimes referred to as self-directed hypnotherapy or autohypnosis, shares many characteristics of relaxation techniques and hypnosis in which someone else induces you into a trance. It has the distinct advantage of not relying on a hypnotist's presence. There is scientific evidence, based on brain wave changes, that you can control pain with self-hypnosis. People who are prone to panic attacks, migraine headaches, some forms of epilepsy, and anxiety, all of which are often accompanied by dizziness, are also helped by self-hypnosis.

Although you can learn relaxation techniques from a book or tape, self-hypnosis requires personal instruction because it is more intense and takes time to learn. If you are willing to make this commitment, find a coach or teacher who is not only an expert in hypnosis but also understands the problems associated with dizziness.

To find a qualified hypnotist, you can ask your physician for a referral or contact one of the societies listed in Appendix A.

Biofeedback

Biofeedback techniques help you to recognize, modify, and control certain involuntary habits or bodily responses, and such techniques can enhance self-hypnosis. They are quite useful for patients who are suffering from dizziness as well as anxiety, tension, and muscle pain, especially symptoms associated with high blood pressure, migraine headaches, cardiac arrhythmias, or epilepsy.

The physician, nurse, mental health professional, or physical therapist who is trained in biofeedback makes use of machines that allow patients to find out about some of the inner workings of their bodies. Biofeedback is a medically safe and painless learning process that uses trial and error, allowing you to consciously control certain functions that are traditionally regarded as purely involuntary.

An electrode is attached to some part of your body—often a finger, palm of the hand, or the skin over a muscle or muscle group. The machine can measure changes in temperature and feed back information about your level of muscle activity and blood flow. It does this with a flashing light-bulb or beep.

The machine yields information but doesn't do anything in itself. However, it serves as an excellent learning tool, because you can make internal adjustments to alter signals. The biofeedback therapist can be described as analogous to a coach, standing at the sidelines giving suggestions on how to change performance.

The goal of biofeedback is often to change patterns of response to stress that cause pain or some other symptom of disease. It can be a fine adjunct to any kind of psychological or physical therapy, helpful for patients who are trying to learn to use muscles differently, or whose dizziness is secondary to anxiety or some other condition.

To find a biofeedback therapist, ask your doctor or contact one of the professional associations listed in Appendix A.

Psychotherapy

If your dizziness has anxiety or depression as the underlying cause, you will certainly want to seek help from someone in the mental health professions (see chapter 7).

Treatment

There are a number of different kinds of psychotherapy available. *Psychoanalysis* helps patients understand and change basic underlying patterns of feelings and behavior that are usually rooted in early development. In psychoanalysis, the patient begins to make that which is unconscious conscious. It usually requires a lengthy commitment of time, and can be costly. *Exploratory or insight psychotherapy* is more goal oriented; in *cognitive therapy*, the sessions may be very interactive, focusing on conscious thoughts that link up external events and emotional responses. It, too, may be goal oriented. *Family therapy* is based on the theory that problems experienced by one person are a reflection of some problem within the family. Thus, all or part of a family meets simultaneously with the therapist. *Group therapy* consists of several people who meet together with one or two therapist co-leaders. Participants can see how they are perceived by others, and often the interaction between members represents feelings experienced outside the group. Any of these therapies may be open-ended in time or prearranged for a brief period of time.

Behavior modification therapy is based on learning theory and can be applied in individual, family, or group settings. It is especially useful for people with specific symptoms such as phobias. The theory behind behavior modification is that since a person learns certain behaviors, these can be unlearned through specific exercises and techniques. This therapy is also useful in controlling general anxieties, pain, and other disorders. Relaxation techniques, exercises, role play, and a number of other modalities, such as bio-feedback or hypnotism are used to change or modify behaviors.

MEDICATION. *Psychopharmacology* is a term used to describe the use of medication to help relieve psychological distress. The medication to treat anxiety and depression has been extremely successful in recent years. Sometimes, even a mild tranquilizer can decrease symptoms of anxiety-related dizziness. Generally, it is used in conjunction with some kind of psychotherapy. Any licensed physician can prescribe medication, but many people feel that it is wise to consult with a psychiatrist, a medical doctor who has specialized training and experience working with drugs and psychological problems. Some psychopharmacologists also offer psychotherapy while others suggest you see another mental health professional. Psychologists and social workers cannot prescribe medication but are trained in counseling.

To find a mental health professional, consult your primary physician or Appendix A.

Helping Yourself

Keeping your life in balance is difficult when your dizziness interferes with daily activities and your attempt to keep a good balance in your personal life.

Explain your situation to those with whom you interact, especially family, friends, and coworkers. Let them know that much of the time you are fine and enjoy a visit to the county fair even if you skip the Ferris wheel. Be honest. Explain that there are times when just looking up and down a supermarket aisle or choosing a book from library shelves can worsen your dizziness.

When Things Are at Their Worst

If you have an acute attack, there are ways to reduce your symptoms. Take these steps:

- Keep your head as still as possible. Lie on a hard surface such as the floor or a firm mattress.
- Remain still until the dizziness and/or nausea stops.
- Without moving your head, move your eyes.
- Then, without moving your head, slowly move your arms and legs.
- If you vomit, wait an hour before trying small sips of water. Then take any medication that your physician has prescribed or recommended, if you are able to keep the water down.
- For the next few hours take precautions against any activity that could cause a fall or accident if you become dizzy again.

Don't Expect Miracles

One of the frustrating things about dizziness is that it comes and goes, sometimes without warning. Even if you are being treated for it, it doesn't go away overnight.

Symptoms may worsen or lessen under certain circumstances or for no reason at all. Your hopes for recovery may be dashed, even though you were overly optimistic that a cure was just around the corner. You may be tempted to change treatment centers. Usually, this won't hasten your recovery; it may mean repeating a number of tests. Time is what you need.

If your dizziness is caused by an associated or underlying medical condition, including hormonal changes or allergies, any exacerbation of those conditions may increase your dizziness. Once they are treated, dizziness should subside.

Take control of your life by following the advice you receive from your physician, physical therapist, dietitian, or others on your team. Pace yourself so you don't get overtired. Don't wait too long to eat or replace fluids.

Take Simple Precautions

Wear the right kind of footwear. Women should avoid high heels. Some people advocate footwear with thick, soft soles for stability, but some studies demonstrate that thin, hard soles offer even more stability. Older people are particularly unstable barefoot.

In your day-to-day activities, try to avoid sudden head turns or position changes. Get out of bed slowly, letting your legs swing over the side even before you sit up. When you arise from a chair or bed, get up slowly, holding on to a steady support and not letting go until you are stable.

When attempting a new activity, entering a hectic situation, or encountering one that has caused problems in the past, ask someone to accompany you. Spend just a brief time there, allowing yourself to become accustomed to it.

To avoid falls when a dizzy spell occurs, keep your home and workplace as safe as possible. Floors should not have thick carpeting or scatter rugs. Bare floors are fine as long as they're not slippery. Encourage family members to keep floors free of shoes, packages, newspapers, toys, and other objects that can be put out of the way. Explain that looking down may be difficult, so you want to be able to count on an obstacle-free route from one place to another.

Chances are that you depend on your visual input to compensate for inner ear problems. Good lighting—day and night—a current eyeglass prescription, and clean glasses will help. Don't carry *anything* that obstructs your view.

Be sure that your shower and bath are safe. Use skid-free mats or strips that are permanently affixed to the bottom. Think about getting a safety rail for the bathtub and a shower stool or chair. This equipment is available at your local surgical supply shop or drugstore.

Daily Routine

Ask someone to help you rearrange your kitchen or office so that things you use regularly don't require lots of bending or reaching. Use a long-handled pole that is constructed to grab things that are too high or too low. Sponges, mops, brooms, and dustpans for the floor should have long handles. Consult a catalog that offers adaptive equipment that can help you go about your routine with the least bending and twisting of your head. These catalogs may be available through a physical or occupational therapist or from your local surgical supply store.

If noise causes dizziness, assess what you can do to avoid exposure at home or work. Earplugs or your own radio and cassette player with earphones may solve this problem.

If crowds bother you and you have trouble focusing, try shopping or going to restaurants at off-hours, when these places are the least crowded. When you feel more confident, try to get back to your old habits and schedules.

Driving

If driving a car is important to you for work, shopping, and errands, or simply as a means to get out of your house, you are undoubtedly wondering: should I drive?

Discuss this with your doctor, but also trust your own judgment. If you are dizzy and unstable on your feet a good deal of the time, you may not want to drive. At least not yet. If you have episodes of dizziness and feel fine between them, you may question the safety of driving. Suppose you're on a highway or freeway and you're suddenly struck with an attack.

Despite your dizziness, you should be able to see well enough to get off the road or at least pull over to the side. If your dizziness is sometimes accompanied by an alteration of consciousness, or if the attacks are blinding, you should drive only where you can easily and quickly pull over.

Night driving or driving on dark, dreary, rainy, or snowy days may be difficult. Impaired vision, rain or snow hitting the windshield, or movement of the wipers may trigger a dizzy spell.

Be prepared to make occasional, unplanned stops. Carry water, snacks, an umbrella, and an extra jacket or raincoat so you can wait out a storm comfortably until you feel better. If your budget permits, consider a car phone.

Ask your physician for a note to carry that attests to your balance disorder. If you should be stopped by the police because your driving is momentarily erratic as you pull over, and you are also experiencing abnormal eye movements (nystagmus), you could be suspected of driving while under the influence of alcohol or other substances. Be aware that many physicians will advise dizzy patients not to drive for months or years without strong reason. Fear of lawsuit is the main reason for the over-cautious approach.

Coping with Uncertainty

Do what you can to help yourself overcome dizziness, including medical treatment, exercise, and the various tips listed previously. Some people feel better just knowing they are doing something to help themselves; others want the health professional to "take over" and cure them.

Unfortunately, dizziness isn't like a broken leg. Doctors can't just fix it or predict when the repair will be complete, even after surgery.

Self-help organizations may have meetings in your community or provide newsletters and names of people whom you can contact by phone. These groups are listed in Appendix A.

Future Hope for Chronic Dizziness

There is still a great deal that medical researchers don't yet know about chronic dizziness—the kind that involves prolonged symptoms. Animal studies can only tell us so much. We can observe imbalance and even come to conclusions about reflexes and physiology behind the vestibular system, but the feeling of dizziness can only be expressed by a human being. Repeated spells of acute dizziness in which the symptoms are of abrupt onset and short duration are usually related to a problem within the ear. More and more, treatments are available for this, and new ones are continually being developed.

Research on dizziness focuses on people and is usually conducted at large universities and medical centers. If you are asked to participate in such a study, by law you should be fully informed about the nature of the study and any associated risks. When you participate in research, you should not be asked to pay for the tests or your care.

If you participate in a study, make sure that you are told the rationale behind it. You should also be assured that you can withdraw from the study at any time without jeopardizing your care with any physician or hospital. Your records and identity should be kept confidential, and you should be treated in a respectful, dignified manner without undergoing anything invasive, including surgery, or any potentially dangerous situation that you do not agree to. Fortunately, there are minimal risks in research for vestibular problems.

Past participants in such research have made it possible to find new, improved ways of treating dizziness. Surgical procedures are improving; physicians are employing new techniques that allow for faster recovery.

New drugs and new combinations of drugs are being developed, and physical therapy is becoming more individualized and more efficient at training people to recover their former functioning. Collaboration between professionals who treat dizziness has led to more innovative therapies and greater coordination of care. Patients are becoming better advocates for themselves, and this, too, results in better care.

The prognosis, then, for most people suffering from dizziness is very promising.

Finding the right doctor isn't always easy. Your own primary care physician should be able to recommend a specialist to you, or you can consult some of the sources listed in Appendix A.

You may learn about a balance or vestibular center from advertisements or friends. Such a center may be helpful if it is located in a larger medical center or complex that you have already learned to respect. But sometimes, these specialized "centers" are not staffed by knowledgeable physicians, administer unnecessary tests, and advocate only a particular treatment. They may even perform needless surgery. For this reason, we suggest that you carefully check out any proposed tests or treatments before undergoing them.

Helpful Sources

The following organizations can be helpful in providing you with information and in recommending a physician or other health care professional. Many can also provide you with free relevant reading material and/or a catalog of booklets, books, and tapes for purchase. Those for whom no telephone number is listed request that you do *not* call but rather send a self-addressed, stamped envelope requesting information and/or referrals. All of the organizations welcome written requests; those with 800 phone numbers are usually prepared to handle requests by telephone.

ALLERGIES
American Academy of Allergy and Immunology
611 East Wells Street
Milwaukee, WI 53202
414-272-6071
1-800-822-ASMA

ARTHRITIS
Arthritis Foundation
P.O. Box 1900
Atlanta, GA 30326
404-872-7100
1-800-283-7800

ATAXIA
National Ataxia Foundation
750 Twelve Oaks Center
15500 Wayzata Boulevard
Wayzata, MN 55391
612-473-7666

BIOFEEDBACK
Association for Applied
Psychophysiology and Biofeedback
10200 West 44th Avenue
Suite 304
Wheat Ridge, CO 80033
303-422-8436

BOOKS ON TAPE
National Library for the
Blind and Physically Handicapped
Library of Congress
1291 Taylor Street, NW
Washington, DC 20542
202-707-5100
1-800-424-8567

Books on tape as well as the appropriate players are available to those who, for any one of many medical reasons, find it difficult or impossible to read.

BRAIN AND CENTRAL DISORDERS
National Institute of Neurological
Disorders and Stroke (NINDS)
9000 Rockville Pike
Building 31, Room 8A16
Bethesda, MD 20892
301-496-5751

Acoustic Neuroma Association
P.O. Box 12402
Atlanta, GA 30355
404-237-8023

National Multiple Sclerosis Society
733 Third Avenue
New York, NY 10017
212-986-3240
1-800-LEARN-MS

Epilepsy Foundation of America
4351 Garden City Drive
Landover, MD 20785
301-459-3700
1-800-EFA-1000

National Stroke Association
8480 East Orchard Road
Suite 1000
Englewood, CO 80111-5015
303-762-9922
1-800-STROKES

DIABETES
American Diabetes Association
P.O. Box 25757
1600 Duke Street
Alexandria, VA 22314
703-549-1500
1-800-232-3472

EAR-RELATED DISORDERS
American Academy of Otolaryngology–
Head and Neck Surgery (AAOHNS)
One Prince Street
Alexandria, VA 22314
703-836-4444

DEAFNESS
American Speech-Language-Hearing Association
10801 Rockville Pike
Rockville, MD 20852
301-897-5700
TDD (telecommunications device for the deaf):
301-897-8682
Voice: 1-800-638-8255

National Institute on Deafness and
Other Communication Disorders (NIDCD)
Information Clearinghouse
1 Communication Avenue
Bethesda, MD 20892-3456
1-800-241-1044
TYY (Teletypewriter): 1-800-241-1055

DIZZINESS
Vestibular Disorders Association (VEDA)
P.O. Box 4467
Portland, OR 97208-4467
503-229-7705

TINNITUS
American Tinnitus Association
P.O. Box 5
Portland, OR 97207-0005
503-248-9985

HEADACHES
National Headache Foundation
5252 N. Western Avenue
Chicago, IL 60625
312-878-7715
1-800-843-2256

HYPNOSIS
The American Society of Clinical Hypnosis
2200 East Devon Avenue
Suite 291
Des Plaines, IL 60018

Society for Clinical and Experimental Hypnosis
128-A Kings Park Drive
Liverpool, NY 13090

MENTAL HEALTH
American Psychiatric Association
Division of Public Affairs
1400 K Street, NW
Washington, DC 20005
202-682-6000

American Psychological Association
750 First Street, NE
Washington, DC 20002-4242
202-336-5500
1-800-374-2721

National Mental Health Association (NHMA)
1021 Prince Street
Alexandria, VA 22314-2971
703-684-7722
1-800-969-NMHA

Information Resources and Inquiries Branch
National Institute of Mental Health (NIMH)
5600 Fishers Lane
Room 7C-02
Rockville, MD 20857

National Association of Social Workers
750 First Street, NE
Suite 700
Washington, DC 20002
301-565-0333
1-800-638-8799

American Association for Marriage and Family Therapy
1100 17th Street, NW
10th Floor
Washington, DC 20036
202-452-0109
1-800-374-2638

NUTRITIONAL COUNSELING
American Dietetic Association
216 West Jackson Boulevard
Suite 800
Chicago, IL 60606-6995
312-899-0040
1-800-745-0775
Consumer Hotline: 1-800-366-1655

PHYSICAL THERAPY
American Academy of Physical Medicine
and Rehabilitation
122 South Michigan Avenue
Suite #1300
Chicago, IL 60603
312-922-9366

SELF-HELP
American Self-Help Clearing House
St. Clare's-Riverside Medical Center
25 Pocono Road
Denville, NJ 07834-2995
1-800-367-6274 (from New Jersey)
201-625-7101 (elsewhere)

National Self-Help Clearinghouse
25 West 43rd Street
Room 620
New York, NY 10036

Suggested Reading

Benson, Herbert. **Beyond the Relaxation Response.** New York: Times Books, 1984.

Benson, Herbert, and Miriam Klipper. **The Relaxation Response.** New York: Avon, 1976.

Benson, Herbert, Eileen M. Steward, and the staff of the Mind/Body Medical Institute of New England, Deaconess Hospital, Harvard Medical School. **The Wellness Book: The Comprehensive Guide to Maintaining Health and Treating Stress-Related Illness.** New York: Carol Publishing Group, 1992.

Biermann, June, and Barbara Toohey. **The Diabetic's Book: All Your Questions Answered.** Third revision. New York: Putnam, 1994.

———. **The Diabetics Total Health Book.** Third edition, revised and expanded. New York: Putnam, 1992.

Dachman, Ken, and John Lyons. **You Can Relieve Pain: How Guided Imagery Can Help You Reduce Pain or Eliminate It Altogether.** New York: Harper & Row, 1990.

Engler, Jack, Daniel Goleman. **The Consumer's Guide to Psychotherapy.** New York: Fireside/Simon & Schuster, 1992.

Gershoff, Stanley N., with Catherine Whitney and the Editorial Board of the Tufts University Diet and Nutrition Letter. **The Tufts University Guide to Total Nutrition.** New York: Harper & Row, 1990.

Gold, Mark. **The Good News About Panic, Anxiety and Phobias.** New York: Villard Books, 1989.

Goleman, Daniel, and Joel Gurin, editors. **Mind/Body Medicine.** Yonkers, N.Y.: Consumer Reports Books, 1993.

Haley, Jay. **Uncommon Therapy.** New York: W.W. Norton, 1987.

Hamilton, Michael, et al. **The Duke University Medical Center Book of Diet and Fitness.** New York: Fawcett Columbine, 1991.

Herbert, Victor, and Genell J. Subak-Sharpe, editors. **The Mount Sinai School of Medicine Complete Book of Nutrition.** New York: St. Martin's Press, 1990.

Kaplan, Andrew S. and Gary Williams, Jr. **The TMJ Book.** New York: Pharos Books, 1988.

Kelly, Sean, and Reid J. Kelly. **Hypnosis: Understanding How It Can Work for You.** Reading, Mass.: Addison-Wesley, 1985.

Larson, David E., editor. **Mayo Clinic Family Health Book.** New York: William Morrow & Company, 1990.

Medical Economics Staff. **The PDR Family Guide to Prescription Drugs.** Montvale, N.J.: Medical Economics Data, 1994.

Moyers, Bill. **Healing and the Mind.** New York: Doubleday, 1993.

Pisetsku, David S., with Susan Flamholz Trien. **The Duke University Medical Center Book of Arthritis.** New York: Fawcett Columbine, 1992.

Solomon, Seymour, and Steven Fraccaro. **The Headache Book.** Yonkers, N.Y.: Consumer Reports Books, 1991.

Spiegel, David. **Living Beyond Limits.** New York: Times Press, 1993.

Surks, Martin I. **The Thyroid Book.** Yonkers, N.Y.: Consumer Reports Books, 1993.

Vernick, David M., Constance Grzelka, and the Editors of Consumer Reports Books. **The Hearing Loss Handbook.** Yonkers, N.Y.: Consumer Reports Books, 1993.

Weill, Andrew. **Natural Health, Natural Medicine: A Comprehensive Manual for Wellness and Self-Care.** Boston: Houghton-Mifflin, 1990.

Young, Stuart, Bruce Dobozin, and Margaret Miner. **Allergies.** Yonkers, N.Y.: Consumer Reports Books, 1992.

Glossary

Acoustic neuroma. A benign brain tumor that arises on a part of the eighth cranial nerve, the nerve that carries information about sound and vestibular function from the ear to the brain.

Aminoglycosides. Antibiotics that include streptomycin and gentamicin, among others. These drugs adversely affect vestibular function, but are sometimes used therapeutically for people with severe dizziness.

Ampulla. Dilated or swollen ends of the semicircular-shaped canals in the inner ear that affect balance.

Anemia. A condition in which there are fewer than the normal number of red blood cells. Anemia includes various forms, and symptoms may include dizziness and imbalance.

Anesthetic. A substance that causes loss of sensation in all or part of the body. Local anesthetic causes lack of sensation in a limited area. General anesthetic causes loss of consciousness and sensation.

Antibiotics. Drugs that can destroy or interfere with the development of certain bacterial infections.

Antihistamines. A group of drugs used to relieve the symptoms of allergies. Antihistamines work by blocking the effects of histamine, an active substance in allergic reactions. Some of these drugs are effective against dizziness.

Anxiety. An uncomfortable, often vague feeling of uneasiness, agitation, or fear, usually resulting either from uncertainty or from a consciously or unconsciously anticipated threatening event or outcome.

Astigmatism. A condition in which the curve of the cornea is uneven, making it difficult to clearly focus on an object and resulting in blurred vision.

Ataxia. A condition in which the ability to coordinate movement is impaired. It may be caused by medications; poor information from eyes, ears, or other parts of the balance system; or a disease of the brain.

Audiogram. A noninvasive test that measures hearing. It consists of two parts: the first measures sounds, the second measures the ability to understand speech.

Auditory. Refers to the sense of hearing.

Auditory brain-stem response (ABR). Sometimes called brain-stem audio evoked responses (BAER) or auditory evoked response, this is a noninvasive test that measures hearing and is especially useful for detecting an acoustic neuroma. It is based on the principle that sounds evoke a characteristic pattern of brain waves.

Auricle. Also called the *pinna*. It is the external ear, the part we can see.

Barotrauma. A condition that sometimes occurs in divers, who may call it "middle ear squeeze." It occurs when air fails to enter the middle ear space and the diver experiences temporary hearing loss and dizziness. Inner ear barotrauma is a more serious condition.

Benign. Mild or nonmalignant; used to describe an illness or growth. A benign tumor does not invade or destroy neighboring normal tissue, nor does it spread to other parts of the body.

Benign paroxysmal positional vertigo (BPPV). A syndrome that consists of episodes of spinning or vertigo and that occurs with particular head positions.

Benign positional vertigo (BPV). *See* Benign paroxysmal positional vertigo.

Biofeedback. A training technique that enables an individual to gain some element of voluntary control over autonomic body functions, such as pulse, skin temperature, and brain wave rhythms. It is based on the principle that a desired response is learned when you receive information or feedback.

Blood count. The number of red cells, white cells, and platelets in a given sample of blood.

Board-certified specialist. A physician who received formal training in a medical or a surgical specialty and then passed the relevant examination.

Body imaging. Examination techniques that give a picture of the body's interior, such as X rays, CT scans, ultrasound, and MRI.

Brain stem. The portion of the brain that performs motor, sensory, and reflex functions.

Bruit. An abnormal sound or murmur heard while a physician is examining and listening to an organ or gland.

Caloric testing. A test that requires irrigation of the ear with hot and/or cold water or air to measure vestibular functions.

Cardiovascular. Referring to circulation, the heart, and the blood vessels. In a cardiovascular medical examination, blood pressure is taken, the heart is listened to with a stethoscope, and other tests may be administered.

Central nervous system. The brain and spinal cord.

Cerebellum. The part of the brain responsible for coordination.

Cerebral atrophy. Deterioration of brain cells that can affect various forms of functioning, including balance and equilibrium.

Cerebral cortex. The thinking and conscious part of the brain.

Cerebral vascular accident (CVA). More commonly known as a *stroke*. A stroke is damage to the brain caused by interruption of blood flow to a part of the brain. There are three kinds: *Thrombotic* stroke consists of a clot forming in the artery, blocking blood flow to the brain; an *embolic* stroke occurs when a piece of clot that originated somewhere other than the brain is carried by the bloodstream to an artery leading to the brain, causing an obstruction; and a *hemorrhagic* stroke occurs when a blood vessel in or near the brain breaks, spilling blood into or around the brain.

Cerebrospinal fluid (CSF). Fluid that flows through and protects the brain.

Cholesteatoma. An abnormal growth of skin tissue in the ear, usually caused by repeated infections.

Chronic. Continuous or of long duration. Certain diseases are chronic in that they slowly progress and/or continue for long periods of time.

Cilia. Hairlike projections on the surface of some cells. They are found in the tiny area of neural tissue in the inner ear.

Cochlea. Part of the inner ear that functions in hearing. It resembles in shape a snail's shell, is lined with tiny hairs, and is filled with two kinds of fluid.

Cochlear aqueduct. A channel through the temporal bone that joins the cochlea to the cerebrospinal fluid (CSF).

Cochleosacculotomy. A surgical procedure performed for Ménière's disease that can relieve pressure in the inner ear.

Compensate. A term often used in discussing patients with dizziness. It refers to the way the brain adjusts to mixed messages from the various parts of the balance system, resulting in the reeducation of the brain or cessation of dizziness.

Complete blood count (CBC). *See* Blood count.

Computerized tomography (CT) scans. A diagnostic technique that uses computers and X rays to obtain highly detailed, three-dimensional information on body tissues as well as bone. Contrast dye is usually injected into the patient prior to the procedure.

Conductive hearing loss. Hearing loss that is caused by an error in the transmission of sound from the outside world to the cochlea.

Cranial nerves. The twelve nerves that originate in the brain, emerging from the skull. Problems with the eighth cranial nerve can cause dizziness. Other cranial nerves can be involved in diseases of the skull base that cause dizziness.

Cupula. Sensory receptors in the ampulla, the dilated or swollen end of the semicircular-shaped canals in the inner ear that are responsible for balance sensation.

Depression. Emotional state characterized by feelings of sadness, despair, and discouragement, which may be either appropriate or out of proportion to reality.

Diabetes. A condition in which the body fails to satisfactorily utilize sugar, starches, and other foods into the energy needed to sustain life.

Disequilibrium. Refers to unsteadiness or imbalance.

Diuretics. Drugs that cause urinary excretion of fluid, sodium, and potassium. Diuretics are used to treat high blood pressure. They are also used to treat Ménière's disease.

Drop attacks. Sudden falls to the ground without loss of consciousness or other symptoms before the fall. This is different from a fainting spell, where there is a loss of consciousness. Drop attacks occur when muscles become weak. They can be caused by a blockage of a particular set of blood vessels in the brain rather than a problem with a set of muscles or a brain disease. They can occur in Ménière's disease.

Dynamic platform posturography. A test that examines all aspects of the balance system by having the subject stand on a platform that may or may not be moved. The subject must change posture and may eventually lose balance.

Eardrum. *See* Tympanic membrane.

Eighth cranial nerve. The nerve coming from the brain that is essential to the senses of hearing and balance. A benign tumor called an *acoustic neuroma* can arise on this nerve.

Electrocardiogram (EKG or ECG). A graphic record or tracing of the action of various portions of the heart. It is the most commonly used noninvasive test of heart function.

Electroencephalogram (EEG). A painless diagnostic test that yields a graphic record measuring electrical activity in various parts of the brain. Commonly used to diagnose seizure disorders.

Electrolytes. Compounds that provide the necessary environment for the body's cells. They include potassium, sodium, and chloride.

Electronystagmography. A battery of tests that assess the relationship between the eyes and the vestibular system, and help diagnose the cause of dizziness.

Encephalitis. An acute inflammatory disease of the brain that is due to a direct attack by a virus or as a complication of another infection.

Endolymph. Fluid that is contained within the sacs and tubes of the inner ear.

Endolymphatic hydrops. An accumulation of the fluid, *endolymph,* within the sacs and tubes of the inner ear. This creates an expansion of the endolymphatic compartment and produces pressure that interferes with the functioning of the inner ear, affecting both hearing and balance.

Endolymphatic sac surgery. Surgical procedure performed for Ménière's disease in which the fluid is drained from the endolymphatic compartment of the inner ear.

Epilepsy. Also known as a seizure disorder. It is not one but an entire group of neurological disorders. It is caused by an uncontrolled electrical discharge from the nerve cells of the cerebral cortex in the brain. Seizures, as attacks of epilepsy are called, are of various types.

Eustachian tube. A narrow tube that slants down from the air space in the middle ear to the back of the nose. The passageway is usually closed, but swallowing or yawning opens it, allowing an exchange of air. This equalizes the air pressure between the middle ear and the outside.

Fistula. An abnormal opening from one internal organ to another or leading to a surface. Fistulas can occur between the inner ear and the middle ear.

Gaze test. A test to determine if spontaneous nystagmus is present when you look in various directions.

Hallpike test. A test to determine if nystagmus occurs during various head positions. It is most useful in the diagnosis of benign positional vertigo.

Hypertension. High blood pressure.

Hyperventilate. A condition in which breathing becomes deep and rapid and too much carbon dioxide is exhaled.

Hypnosis. A passive, trancelike state resembling normal sleep, during which perception and memory are altered, permitting the person to respond to suggestions then or during a posthypnotic period. Self-hypnosis (also called autohypnosis, self-directed hypnotherapy) shares characteristics with relaxation techniques and hypnosis, but doesn't require a hypnotist for induction.

Hypotension. Low blood pressure.

Incus. One of the three bones of hearing (ossicles), found in the oval window.

Inner ear. *See* Labyrinth.

Inner ear fluids. *See* Endolymph *and* Perilymph.

Labyrinth. The inner ear, consisting of a complex system of chambers and passageways. It is encased in an odd-shaped, complicated bone called the temporal bone, one of many bones of the skull.

Labyrinthectomy. A surgical procedure in which the labyrinth and, therefore, all hearing and balance function in the ear are destroyed. Often performed for Ménière's disease and other vestibular disorders involving the ear.

Labyrinthitis. A term that describes several different disorders of the labyrinth. They can be caused by bacteria or a virus, and can lead to severe vertigo and hearing loss. The term is commonly misused and applied to any vague dizziness that is not understood.

Lesion. A lump, abscess, or mass of cells. It can be benign or cancerous.

Lumbar puncture. *See* Spinal tap.

Maculae. Tiny areas of neural tissue in the saccule and utricle of the inner ear, containing cells with hairlike projections called cilia. The maculae are important for the body to sense the direction of gravity.

Magnetic resonance imaging (MRI). A diagnostic technique that produces a three-dimensional, cross-sectional image and can detect dead or degenerating cells, blockage of blood flow, and other abnormalities in the body. These abnormalities might include tumors, stroke, and various diseases or lesions in the brain.

Malleus. One of the ossicles, the three small bones of hearing in the middle ear. It is attached to the eardrum as well as to another hearing bone, the incus.

Membranous labyrinth. A network of three fluid-filled, thin layers of tissue in the inner ear.

Ménière's disease. A combination of symptoms that include repeated episodes of vertigo, ringing in the ear, feeling of fullness in the ear, and often hearing loss.

Meningitis. A viral or bacterial infection of the membranes covering the brain and spinal cord. Symptoms are usually acute, and may include dizziness.

Middle ear. Part of the ear that reaches from the eardrum to the bone of the skull. It is an air-filled space or cavity that also contains the ossicles, the three bones of hearing.

Migraine. A recurring headache, thought to arise from problems within the small arteries that go to the brain. It is characterized by a number of symptoms, including warning symptoms that precede it. Dizziness may occur prior to or during an attack.

Migraine equivalent. A recurring disorder in which someone may have bouts of vertigo, hearing loss, and tinnitus, but only occasionally (if ever) develop a headache.

Mild turning. A less severe form of vertigo in which a person can still function normally in every way. It may be a sign of a mild ear dysfunction but can also be serious and should be reported to a physician if it persists.

Ministroke. *See* Transient ischemic attack.

Motion sickness. A feeling of nausea and/or dizziness that overcomes someone when he or she is moving, usually in a car, boat, or airplane. Another kind of motion sickness is caused when one is still but one's surroundings are rotated or swayed.

Multiple sclerosis (MS). A disease of the central nervous system characterized by such symptoms as weakness, numbness in arms or legs, blurred vision, imbalance, and unsteadiness in walking. Nystagmus is often present in MS.

Multisensory dizziness. A generalized dizziness that seems to have many causes rather than just one. It is most often found in older people or in those with diabetes.

Myringotomy. A surgical procedure in which an incision is made into the eardrum to drain an acutely infected ear. A tiny hollow tube may be inserted into the eardrum, allowing continuous draining of fluid. The tube is called a tympanostomy tube.

Neurologist. A physician who specializes in disorders of the nervous system.

Neurosurgeon. A physician who performs surgery on the brain, spinal cord, or peripheral nerves.

Nystagmus. An abnormal series of jerky eye movements, usually horizontal but also occurring in up-and-down, rotary, or oblique directions.

Ocular dizziness. Dizziness caused by a problem with the eyes.

Ophthalmologist. A physician who specializes in the treatment and surgery of the eyes.

Ophthalmoscope. A devise with a light and mirror used to examine the inside of the eye.

Optokinetic system. A reflex that causes the eyes to move when the field of vision moves.

Orthostasis. *See* Postural hypotension.

Oscillopsia. An illusion that stationary objects are moving back and forth or up and down.

Ossicles. The three small bones of hearing, found in the middle ear. *See also* Incus, Malleus, *and* Stapes.

Otititis media. An acute, usually painful ear infection of the middle ear.

Otolaryngologist. A physician who specializes in the treatment and surgery of the ear, nose, and throat.

Otolithic membrane. A gelatinous mass in which the otoliths are located.

Otolith organs. One of the two types of organs of balance in the inner ear. The otolith organs are called the saccule and utricle.

Otoliths. Crystals of calcium carbonate in the inner ear that shift their weight according to gravity or due to movements occurring in a straight line.

Otosclerosis. A hardening and new formation of bone in the middle ear that can cause hearing loss and ringing in the ears.

Otoscope. An instrument with a light, magnifying lens, and tip that a physician can carefully insert into the ear as far as the eardrum. The otoscope permits examination of the external ear, the eardrum, and, through the eardrum, the bones of the middle ear.

Oval window. The oval-shaped opening to the cochlea, the hearing portion of the inner ear.

Panic disorder. A disorder characterized by sudden, severe, unprovoked terror. Disabling attacks are accompanied by irrational fears and symptoms that can resemble a heart attack. Dizziness and faintness may also accompany it.

Paroxysmal. Sudden, episodic, and usually brief.

Perilymph. Fluid found in the outer two compartments of the cochlea of the inner ear.

Perilymph fistula. An opening between the middle ear and the part of the inner ear that contains perilymph fluid. It permits fluid from the inner ear to leak out into the middle ear.

Peripheral vestibular system. *See* Vestibular apparatus.

Periphery. In discussing the balance system, refers to the ears, eyes, muscles, and joints. The other part of the balance system consists of the central nervous system (brain and spinal cord).

Phobia. Terror, dread, or panic at the thought, sight, or confrontation with something such as an object, situation, or activity.

Pinna. *See* Auricle.

Platform fistula test. A test done on a moving platform that determines body sway and yields information regarding how the middle ear responds to pressure.

Postural hypotension. A frequent cause of dizziness, the term refers to the sudden dropping of blood pressure when someone stands or sits up.

Presyncope. A feeling of faintness that comes on quickly and is brief, without loss of consciousness, as in fainting.

Proprioceptive system. The receptor/processing system that delivers information to the brain from the ears, eyes, muscles, and joints.

Pursuit system. The system that keeps vision fixed on an object when it moves slowly across the field of vision.

Recurrent vestibulopathy. A condition that closely resembles Ménière's disease, but with shorter spells of vertigo and a tendency to improve.

Relaxation techniques. Various techniques that can reduce emotional stress and physical symptoms. Passive relaxation is similar to self-hypnosis or meditation. Progressive relaxation also includes the tensing and relaxing of specific muscle groups.

Rotary testing. Tests of the vestibular system that make use of rotary movement. Either the patient's chair is moved or his or her head is moved.

Round window. Opening in the cochlea that vibrates in the opposite direction of the oval window, permitting a minute flow of fluid in the cochlea. This allows transmission of sound by way of vibrations.

Saccade and calibration tests. Tests that accurately measure the speed of the eye movement in electronystagmography.

Saccule. A chamber of the inner ear containing otoliths that detect linear movements in the vertical plane and gravity when a person is in an upright position.

Scopolamine. A drug that is helpful in preventing motion sickness. It is most often prescribed as a patch, which allows the medication to be absorbed through the skin.

Semicircular canals. Inner-ear balancing structure that measures angular motion.

Sensorineural hearing loss. Hearing loss that usually arises from an abnormality of the cochlea hair cells or the auditory nerve. Some people are born with it, while others develop it in childhood or adulthood. Certain medications and exposure to loud and continuous noises can also cause it.

Skull. Bony framework of the head, covering the brain and supporting the face.

Somatization. The experience of unconsciously expressing a psychological conflict or need in a number of vague, multiple, and physical symptoms for which no physical cause is found, despite an extensive medical evaluation. Dizziness often plays an important role in these symptoms. *Somatizers* are persons who often suffer from a form of depression that is treatable.

Sonogram. A computer picture that uses ultrasound (high-frequency sound waves) to examine the position, form, and function of anatomical structures. A sonogram is also the record of these ultrasound tests.

Spinal tap. Removal of fluid from the spinal column in order to reveal information about the brain and spinal cord. Also called *lumbar puncture*.

Stapedectomy. Surgical removal of all or part of the stapes, it can restore hearing when otosclerosis has developed in one ear and the stapes fail to vibrate properly.

Stapes. One of the three small bones of hearing, found in the oval window of the inner ear.

Snycope. Fainting or passing out with loss of consciousness.

Syphilis. A disease caused by a spiral-shaped bacterium (spirochete) spread during sexual contact. It can also be passed on by a mother to her unborn child. Dizziness and balance problems can exist, with or without other symptoms, in someone with untreated syphilis.

Systemic disease. A disease that affects the whole body rather than just one portion of it.

Tack operation. A surgical procedure done for Ménière's disease, in which a metal tack is placed through the foot plate of the stapes bone into the inner ear.

Temporal bone. The part of the skull in which the inner ear is located.

Temporomandibular joint disorders (TMJ). Problems with the jaw joint and its muscles, often resulting in pain in the jaw, head, or any area in between. Dizziness and ringing in the ears may also be associated with TMJ.

Thyroid gland. A gland located at the base of the neck that wraps around the windpipe. Both an overactive and underactive thyroid can cause a number of symptoms, among them mild dizziness and, in some instances, sensorineural hearing loss.

Tinnitus. Tingling or ringing in one or both ears.

Tumor. A swelling or enlargement in the body, it can be either benign (noncancerous) or malignant (cancerous).

Transient ischemic attack (TIA). Symptoms caused by a brief episode of insufficient blood flowing to the brain or a part of the brain.

Tympanic membrane. Another term for the eardrum, the structure separating the ear canal from the middle ear air cavity.

Tympanostomy tubes. Tubes that are surgically placed into the eardrum to permit an infected ear to drain.

Utricle. The organ in the inner ear that detects gravity or linear movements in the horizontal plane of the head.

Vertigo. An illusion of rotation, a feeling that either you or the world around you is spinning. Usually caused by a problem in the inner ear that leads to conflicting information being sent to the brain.

Vestibular apparatus. The balance part of the inner ear, adjacent to the cochlea and connected by channels. Its function is to maintain equilibrium and balance. It is sometimes called the *peripheral vestibular system, vestibular organs,* or *vestibular structures.*

Vestibular aqueduct. Sometimes called an endolymphatic duct, it is a soft tissue connecting the endolymph-containing portion of the inner ear and the endolymphatic sac.

Vestibular nerve. The nerve between the ear and the brain that carries information relating to body orientation to the brain.

Vestibular nerve section. A surgical procedure in which the vestibular nerve is cut, bringing significant relief from spells of vertigo but often leaving some mild imbalance symptoms.

Vestibular neuronitis. Thought to be an inflammation of the vestibular nerve, it causes vertigo, dizziness, and vomiting, and often follows a viral infection. It can lie dormant and recur later.

Vestibulo ocular reflex. A reflex consisting of eye movements evoked by stimulation of the vestibular system.

Vestibular organs. *See* Vestibular apparatus.

Vestibular structures. *See* Vestibular apparatus.

Vestibular suppressants. Drugs that have sedative properties and can suppress the vestibular system, reducing the severity of dizziness.

Vestibular system. The collection of neural elements that work together to detect movement and position. It consists of the brain and the parts of the inner ear (the vestibular apparatus) that are motion sensors.

Work-up. The combined results of a medical examination and tests used to arrive at a diagnosis and complete medical picture.

Index

Bold typeface denotes word definitions.
Italic typeface denotes figures.

80 - Abnormal level of certain chemical
(calcium - sodium - Potassium in the Blood)

30 -
65 - ENG - (a number of but

(86) ✗✗
✗ 154
160 -
161 - Niacin

CPSIA information can be obtained
at www.ICGtesting.com
Printed in the USA
LVHW031607150720
660781LV00002B/278